The Heart OF THE Matter

The Heart

OF THE Matter

THE THREE KEY BREAKTHROUGHS TO PREVENTING HEART ATTACKS

Peter Salgo, M.D.

■ WITH JOE LAYDEN ■

WM

WILLIAM MORROW
An Imprint of HarperCollins*Publishers*

The names and identifying details of each
of the patients mentioned in this book have been
changed to preserve patient confidentiality.

HarperCollins books may be purchased for educational,
business, or sales promotional use. For information please write:
Special Markets Department, HarperCollins Publishers Inc.,
10 East 53rd Street, New York, NY 10022.

FIRST EDITION

Designed by Adrian Leichter

Printed on acid-free paper

Library of Congress Cataloging-in-Publication Data

Salgo, Peter.
    The heart of the matter : the three key breakthroughs to
preventing heart attacks / Peter Salgo, with Joe Layden.
        p.   cm.
    ISBN 0-06-054428-7
    1. Coronary heart disease—Prevention—Popular works.
I. Layden, Joe.   II. Title.

RC685.C6S26   2004
616.1'2305—dc22

                                    2003061444

04   05   06   07   08   WBC/RRD   10   9   8   7   6   5   4   3   2   1

For Heidi

You changed my book and my life
and made them both better

Contents

■ ■ ■

CONTENTS

Acknowledgments

■ ■ ■

I have had the great good fortune of working closely with some of the most talented physicians of our time. Many have given me the benefit of their extraordinary knowledge, experience, and judgment. Quite a few have endured long discussions in hospital corridors, cafeterias, and nurses' stations without complaint. Doctors Jerry Gliklich, Robert Heissenbuttel, Donald Landry, Sun Hi Lee, Frank Livelli, Anne Peters, LeRoy Rabbani, Stefano Ravalli, James Reiffel, David Sherman, Brian Scully, Stanley Schneller, Alan Schwartz, Joseph Tenenbaum, Byron Thomashow, and Mark Warshofsky managed to help me while maintaining their grace, good humor, and unfailing dedication to clear constructive thought.

My fellow intensive care unit (ICU) specialists have always been available to help when I needed time to prepare this book. For that I am truly grateful. Doctors Arthur Atchabahian, Tricia Brentjens, Debbie Cooper, Terri Koch, Hugh Playford, Robert Sladen, Gebhard Wagener, and Staffan Wahlander have never been less than gracious. They are the best team of physicians with whom it has been my pleasure to work.

Dr. Margaret Wood, Chair of Anesthesiology at New York Presbyterian Hospital, has been generous with her time and flexible in her requests.

Dr. Christine Lesch came to the rescue with crucial research help at just the right time.

And then there is Dr. Desmond Jordan. A friend, and a superb clinician, scholar, and teacher, Desmond volunteered not only his time and energy to this project, but his entire family as well. To Lauren Jordan, Kristin Jordan, and their friend Rebecca Altneu, thank you for your dedication to some rather tedious, but absolutely essential tasks.

Without Eric Gumin this book might never have seen the light of day. It is a small world indeed. For your faith in the project and for your help, thank you.

I have had the pleasure of working with my broadcast agent, Carole Cooper, for more than two decades. A friend and a partner, Carole has supported this project from its inception.

Frank Weimann of the Literary Group gave his wry wit and boundless energy to the effort of making this book a reality.

To Henry Ferris, Debbie Stier, and Suzanne Balaban of HarperCollins, my heartfelt thanks. It is a pleasure working with consummate professionals. What's more, you have made the process fun.

I cannot imagine a better writing partner than Joe Layden. He is tireless, talented, and enthusiastic. He is a reservoir of common sense, insightful questions, and literary skill. Working with Joe has been a treat. Thank you.

From a Chinese Parable

■ ■ ■

One day the emperor summoned to his palace the most famous doctor in all of China and asked the healer a question: "Who is the greatest doctor in our land?" No fool this emperor, for here he was, face-to-face with the most famous doctor in his country, but clearly he, the emperor, was able to make the distinction between fame and greatness. So he had asked a very subtle question, perhaps with the hope of tricking the doctor. But the doctor was no fool, either, and he answered as follows:

"I see people at death's door, in their most dire moments. I operate on them, I draw blood from them. Occasionally I bring them back from the brink of death. And I am the most famous doctor in all of China."

At this, the emperor nodded.

"But I have an older brother," the doctor continued, "and my older brother sees people who are not quite as sick. He sees the earliest forms of their illnesses. He is able to intervene before they knock at death's door, and he saves far more people than I. And he is famous in my village."

Again, the emperor nodded.

"But I have an older brother still, older than he," the doctor added, "and he sees the conditions in our country that make our people sick. He changes these conditions before the people become ill. He has saved millions of lives."

The emperor cocked an eyebrow as the doctor paused.

"And this man, the oldest of my brothers, is well known in my family," the doctor finally said. "So I ask you, Emperor, to tell me: Who is the greatest doctor in all of China?"

At this, the emperor merely smiled and nodded.

The Heart OF THE Matter

CHAPTER ONE

The Heart of the Matter

Something new has happened. There is a buzz in the air in medical meetings all across the country. It's a familiar and wonderful feeling. Where we are with heart disease in the year 2003 is the same place we were with infectious diseases just before the discovery of penicillin, where we were with dentistry just before the advent of fluoridation, where we were with polio on the eve of the Salk vaccine—which is to say, we are on the cusp of an enormous breakthrough. We are about to treat people for heart attack before they get sick. We are about to prevent them from dying. This is the work of the oldest brother in the Chinese parable.

After the widespread introduction of fluoridated water, tooth decay all but disappeared as an American health problem. I'm told dental income (for general practitioners, of course) dropped precipitously, and that's why today everyone seems to be an orthodontist. With any luck it's going to be the same with cardiac specialists. I run a cardiac surgery intensive care unit (ICU). Follow the program in this book and you can put me out of business. That's okay. In fact, I'd be thrilled. I've seen enough damage. I've seen enough people die before their time.

There are two distinct parts to *The Heart of the Matter:* the premise and the promise.

The premise is this: Nobody has ever fully understood what causes heart attacks. It's surprising but true. And because we didn't understand what caused them, we couldn't really get a handle on how to prevent them. All that has changed radically and recently. The past few years have seen an explosion of research papers and presentations confirming the new heart attack theory. We now know what causes heart attacks. The answer is probably going to surprise you (it certainly surprised most doctors). And because we know what causes them, we know how to protect you from them. I will show you what you need to do. It's an amazingly simple and straightforward program.

Through an astounding stroke of good fortune, our new understanding of heart attacks has occurred at the same time when we have found new medicines that can target the heart attack mechanism precisely and powerfully. Our understanding has also led us to use older medications in new ways, to turn off the heart attack mechanism.

The promise is this: Ours will be the last generation to die of premature heart disease in this country.

Bold talk? Not really. In this book you'll find an easily administered self-test—so that you can assess your own susceptibility to heart disease—as well as a formula for beating the disease and a clear, concise explanation for why this formula will work.

To understand how excited I am about this new program, you need to "walk a mile in my shoes" and see heart disease as I have seen it during my career. By training I am an internist and an anesthesiologist. That makes me an intensivist. My specialty is cardiac care. As a director of the open heart intensive care unit at Columbia Presbyterian Hospital in New York, I witness daily the destruction wrought by heart disease. I see the devastation and debris caused by the major killer known to humankind, and it sickens me.

Each day as I make rounds I see the shattered lives and devastated hopes and dreams of people who are just like you and me. They have wives, husbands, children; they have plans. They have wept at weddings, cheered at football games; they have spilled food on the Thanksgiving tablecloth. Now they are at the brink of death. They depend upon ventilators to breathe. They depend upon powerful medications to circulate their blood. Many will not survive. When people do not take care of themselves, or their bodies malfunction despite their best intentions, I see the sad results: patients who need heart transplants, artificial hearts, open heart surgery; patients who are desperately ill.

I see people like Jose Rodriguez, who told me one day through a weary, postsurgical smile that he now knew what it felt like to have an elephant sit on his chest. Two days later, despite the love of his family and the best efforts of medical science, Jose was dead.

People like Josephine Smith, who showed up in the ICU a few hours after collapsing in the produce aisle of her local A & P. Or Howard Martin, a man in his late forties whose weekly round of golf was interrupted by a massive coronary. Imagine the shock! You're out on a sun-splashed par five in the middle of the afternoon, and the next thing you know, you're hooked up to a heart-lung bypass machine. It's that traumatic, that disturbing.

I have seen too much of this. I speak to patients, and I hear a familiar story: "Everything was fine, and then all of a sudden, I got this pain." I speak to families and I hear it again: "He was such an active, vigorous man. Now look at him. I don't know how I'm going to get through this."

As I spoke to those patients who could speak, and as I sought to comfort the families of those who might die, I became angry. I didn't know where to direct my anger, at first. It seemed easy to blame the victims. After all, they had smoked or eaten fatty food or rarely exercised. Eventually I realized anger wasn't going to get me anywhere. If I wanted to help my patients, I needed to focus on the real culprit: the disease itself. As I read the latest reports from the labs and went to conferences across the country, I began to see that something was changing rapidly. I saw optimistic news appearing in forums that usually offered only gloom and doom.

The good news—and believe me, there is *remarkably* good news—is that we now have the ability to prevent you from dying before your time. Am I promising to "save your life"? Well, yes, in a manner of speaking, although I find that phrase to be a bit misleading, because, ultimately, nobody is saved—we all die someday. But I can assure you that this book will vastly improve the quality of your life and give you many more good years on this beautiful planet. Heard that one before? Maybe so. But I'm not talking about some new-age psychobabble designed merely to give you peace of mind, a better outlook on life, and thinner thighs in thirty days. I'm talking about extending your life by as much as twenty to thirty years. I can tell you, in good faith and good conscience, there is absolutely no reason for you to die of premature heart disease.

.....

Mind you, this is not just the opinion of one battled-scarred ICU doc. My program represents a synthesis of information, a patient-friendly approach to something that has been reported over and over again at traditionally staid academic meetings in which participants typically snore themselves to death. Some of the most respected physicians and scientists in the world are willing to go on record saying there is something out there that had never been available before that can save your life. When they speak to me off the record, the conservatives in the academic community are behind me, too—in more ways than one. They support me, because they know there are studies to back up what I'm saying. But pure academics are naturally cautious about speaking to the public, so they're unwilling to go as far as I've gone in this book. I'm advocating a dramatic shift in the treatment of premature heart disease, and a program of preventive maintenance that includes not only traditional guidelines covering diet and exercise (sorry, couch potatoes and potato chip lovers, I'm not letting you off the hook), but a blanket recommendation that adults—even many young adults—embrace pharmacological assistance in the pursuit of longer, healthier lives.

In recent years there has been a lot of nibbling at the edges of a breakthrough in the treatment of coronary heart disease. Although this trend has at times been encouraging, it's also led to a bit of confusion. You hear the diet and nutrition experts say, "We can reduce your risk of heart disease by putting you on the Pritikin diet and lowering the amount of fat you ingest." Then you hear other doctors say, "Well, eating less fat is all well and good, but we've seen no evidence that the Pritikin diet changes the plaque in your arteries, and we all know that plaque causes heart attacks, so Pritikin is full of garbage!"

As it turns out, both points of view are at least partly correct. What was missing for the longest time was the key that unlocks the central mystery of heart disease, and heart attack in particular.

That's why I'm so excited about this new research. It offers the key to beating premature death. The key is simple, elegant, and easy to understand. Everyone deserves access to it. Everyone can turn the key and open the door to a better life.

I'm going to give you the recipe for preventing this disease. What are the ingredients? First of all, lower your cholesterol level. You've heard that before, too, right? Uh-uh. I'm talking about lowering your cholesterol to a level you've never imagined. Forget about 220. Forget about 200 or 185. I'm talking about 180—maybe lower. For everyone! Realistically, the only way this is going to happen is through medication, specifically through the use of a class of drugs known as *statins*, also known as "fat busters," which can pound the body's cholesterol level into submission. Second, we're going to use aspirin therapy, and not merely because of its long-recognized blood-thinning properties. No, for reasons that will be discussed in detail, I'm advocating aspirin therapy to reduce inflammation in the blood vessels that feed the heart (suffice it to say that inflammation is the missing piece of the coronary heart disease puzzle). Finally, there is a strong suggestion that nearly everyone should be treated for a particular infectious disease that is causing heart attacks. I'm talking about *Chlamydia pneumoniae*. Not to be confused with the sexually transmitted disease known popularly as chlamydia, chlamydia pneumonia is a quiet, often symptom-free upper respiratory infection that is pervasive in our society.

It is oddly and alarmingly prevalent among people who have heart attacks.

Again, I'm not throwing a dart into the dark here—there are statistically significant studies demonstrating that people who have heart attacks are more likely to test positive for chlamydia pneumonia; believe me, it's no great stretch to suggest that if you have, or have had, chlamydia pneumonia, you are at much greater risk for a heart attack, and in this book I will explain precisely why.

There seems to be no other infectious disease that fits the profile. For some reason, when we look at the coronary arteries in heart disease patients we often find *C. pneumoniae*. Why? I don't know. Why does pneumococcus like the lungs? Why does *Escherichia* (*E. coli*) like the bowel? Why does *C. pneumoniae* like the arteries of the heart? *It just does*.

That's the foundation of the program: statin therapy, an aspirin a day, elimination of chlamydia pneumonia. There's absolutely no reason not to exercise and eat right, of course, because such behavior is bound to improve the quality of your life, and what's the point of living to be a hundred if you're going to be a big blubber butt who is unable to get around? You need to keep the rest of the machine operating properly so that you don't rust out early.

But let me be clear about this: As effective as diet and exercise are in maintaining a healthy cardiovascular system, this program is a quantum leap better. For years now, everyone has been in the gym, working like crazy, riding bikes, logging miles on the treadmill, pumping tons of iron and steel. They've all been cutting down on their cholesterol and they've thrown away the cigarettes. That's all fine. In fact, it's great. It's like taking a hammer to heart disease. But this formula—a daily, lifelong regimen of aspirin therapy, statin therapy, and periodic testing for and treatment of C. pneumonia—is the equivalent of a sledge-hammer.

Remember how a few decades ago, we all brushed our teeth like crazy, and we still got cavities. Not until fluoride was added to public water supplies did we see the virtual eradication of tooth decay. Does that mean you shouldn't brush your teeth, that you should simply drink fluoridated water? Of course not. It means, sometimes, mere diligence isn't enough.

Medical science has tried everything to beat heart disease: diet, exercise, surgery, angioplasty. Although matters have im-proved, we're still losing the war. Since we've been applying the latest and most innovative techniques available to combating the disease as we know it, it stands to reason that our knowledge has been insufficient to get the job done right. Too many ques-tions have gone unanswered: How can someone with a "clean" angiogram finding still get a heart attack? Why is bypass sur-gery more effective in treating angina than in preventing heart attacks? Can aspirin prevent heart attacks, and, if so, how does it work?

All of these questions, and many more, will be answered in *The Heart of the Matter*, so that you'll have a clear understand-ing of why it's so important to embrace my program. I want you to be informed and enlightened. I want you to feel smarter when you finish this book. I want you to feel confident that this formula can extend your life. God knows that isn't always the case with books about health and medicine. I know readers have been inundated with information in recent years, most of it either misguided or painfully obvious. They've heard every diet doctor in the world shout "My diet (or exercise program) is the best! It'll save your life!" But what is the proof? Most di-ets—the good ones, anyway—are based on common sense.

They *sound like* good ideas. We'll examine some of them later in this book. The results may surprise you. Not only does my formula sound like a good idea, but it has solid research to back it up. The scientific and research communities have often dismissed diet and exercise advocates because they couldn't prove their theories. Critics of the diet gurus pointed to people like Jim Fixx, author of the 1977 best-seller *The Complete Book of Running*, who ate a sensible diet, ran marathons, looked great—and dropped dead at the age of fifty-two. They pointed to Winston Churchill, who ate a lousy diet, drank port wine, smoked cigars, looked like hell—and lived into his nineties.

My thesis is this: We can take the Jim Fixxes of the world and give them the life span of the Winston Churchills—people who live into their eighties and nineties, even if their genes are bad, even if their bodies are producing gobs of bad cholesterol. We've never been able to say that before; what's more, we're beginning to prove it.

If this is so, you may be asking, Then why haven't we heard more about it? Fair question. Pieces of the puzzle have been out there for a while, backed up by scientific research and reported in various publications (significantly, it should be noted, many of these publications were dedicated to specialties other than cardiology). But no one has synthesized the information in this way for you, the person who needs to use the information to prolong your life. Only an omnivorous consumer of medical literature could put the puzzle together.

My background has allowed me to look at premature coronary heart disease from a unique perspective. I'm informed by different sources: my work at the hospital, where I see the damage each day; my work as a journalist (Emmy Award–winning Health and Science correspondent for WCBS-TV, the CBS television network affiliate in New York for more than two decades, and anchor at CNBC); and my work as an academic. I see more reports from more different specialties than any other doctor I know, and I have learned to probe and question the status quo in ways that make other members of the medical establishment uncomfortable. I attend lots of medical conferences, and what I typically see is a group of people talking about their own narrow specialties. But because my experience is so diverse, I go to so many different conferences and hear from so many different specialties, I have a unique vantage point and can consider input and theories from many difference sources.

And so it was that one day, after I had attended a string of conferences (including those hosted by the American Heart Association and the American Diabetes Association), a lightbulb went on in my mind. Suddenly I understood what was happening, and why so many people were dying of premature coronary heart disease; why all of our best efforts to rescue these people were failing. It became apparent to me that there were three clear pieces to the puzzle: an anti-inflammatory piece, an antibiotic piece, and, most important of all, an anticholesterol piece.

One of my pet peeves with the medical and research establishments (including the Food and Drug Administration) is that they often move too slowly. In this case, in which the therapy is relatively harmless and the potential benefits enormous, speed would seem to be of the essence. In fact, by insisting on the accumulation of overwhelming indisputable scientific proof before committing themselves to a recommendation, they are potentially condemning an entire generation to premature death. I've seen articles lately in which some physicians and government officials have been quoted as saying, "Maybe we should be waiting a little longer to prescribe statins." Well, that's just great. If these naysayers are wrong, then the people who might have used statins but didn't are out of luck, because they'll already be dead. That's unacceptable to me. I have crept far out on a limb on this one because I believe it's worth the risk.

Traditional therapy is failing America! The traditional tools that doctors use to prevent heart attacks are not working. That alone provides powerful evidence that we have to rethink our approach. We have to use our new knowledge right now.

For example, look at angioplasty. Doctors are inserting a stent (a small plastic tube) into a patient's damaged coronary artery to increase the flow of blood through it. It sounds like a reasonable approach if you believe (and this is the standard theory) that clogged arteries cause heart attacks. Coronary arteries feed the heart. Damaged, plugged up arteries don't feed the heart well enough. The stent should pry the arteries open again and make the heart healthier. It's logical. It makes perfect sense. There's just one problem: Unless you start taking aspirin and statins after the procedure, it doesn't work well. More than half of unmedicated patients experience another coronary event within two years of having this procedure. The fact that many stents don't work well unless you add medications to the program can't be explained by the old theory of heart disease. Again, this is a powerful hint that the standard model for heart attack is wrong.

The stent isn't the answer. Mechanical repairs to a terminally damaged artery aren't the answer. They aren't the answer because simple mechanical obstruction of a coronary artery by fat, by calcium, by plaque isn't the problem. That is the missing piece of the puzzle: We've been trying to fix the wrong problem! The old theory of heart attack isn't just wrong, it's dangerously wrong. That's what this book is about.

The problem is not gradual obstruction of coronary arteries by debris. It is *inflammation*. Inflammation is an active disease process in the walls of the arteries themselves. This process produces damage that leads to heart attacks. To prevent heart attacks, then, you don't simply reline the arteries with plastic; you turn off the inflammation process that's causing all the trouble. We know how to do this. You do this with statins and aspirin therapy, and perhaps antibiotics (yes, antibiotics for some people with heart disease!). The trick is to start these medications early, before you get sick, and before inflammation has caused lethal damage to your arteries.

As I see it, the greatest challenge in beating heart disease is convincing people to "get with the program." No one likes taking pills. Human nature is such that many people seek treatment only when illness becomes so severe as to be debilitating. If you feel good, you just sort of float along. Unfortunately, in the case of heart disease, it's not at all unusual to feel *great*—right up until the moment you keel over.

But there are plenty of things people do to stay young and feel good. Why do people go to gyms? Why do they eat bran flakes? Is it an enormous leap from eating bran flakes to popping an aspirin once a day? Lots of people don't think so. You'd be shocked at the number of perfectly healthy people in their thirties who take an aspirin a day to keep themselves heart attack–free. They were doing this before we knew that it works. Now we not only know that aspirin can reduce your heart attack risk, but we also know why it works. It's only a matter of time before people use statins the same way.

My program is less a treatment than a commitment to changing your body's chemical processes for life—a *long* life, I should add. When should you make this commitment? Earlier rather than later. Perhaps as early as thirty for the general population, and certainly in the twenties for people who are at greater risk of heart disease, such as diabetics. For those whose father and grandfather died of a heart attack in his thirties? Those people should be on statins from the time they hit junior high school.

Is this radical? You bet it is. The goal is to prevent heart disease from gaining a foothold in your body, and the disease starts early. In some people it's already at work in the teen years. So the only way to beat it is to start attacking the problem at an early age. I realize I'm challenging the medical paradigm. In the past people often waited until disease took root before seeking treatment. Then they saw a doctor who ran a battery of tests and treated the disease. The treatments were complicated, dangerous, and often relatively ineffective. The doctors they saw were, in effect, the youngest of the three doctors in the ancient Chinese parable, famous, courageous, but not quite the best in the kingdom.

I envision a day, in the not-too-distant future, when nearly everyone will be on this program. Only those who experience side effects (a fraction of the population) will be put through a round of tests (we devote an entire chapter to testing later in this book). Those who are tested and are found to have heart disease will have two choices: continue treatment and deal with the side effects, or stop the treatment and risk the consequences, the most obvious and serious of which is death.

We'll address the side effects of statin therapy in detail in this book. There are risks, of course, as there are with any medication. It is my belief, however, that statin therapy is extremely safe for the overwhelming majority of the population, despite the litany of alarming side effects recited during television commercials for the drugs. It's worth noting that if a similar standard were applied to aspirin, the advertisement might sound something like this: "If you start bleeding from your mouth, nose, or ears, please call your doctor." The truth is, if aspirin were presented to the U.S. Food and Drug Administration (FDA) today, I'm not at all sure it would gain approval. And yet aspirin is saving a lot of lives and alleviating a lot of pain. The same is true of statins.

What I advocate is a public-health approach to heart disease. Although this method may be aggressive, it's not unprecedented. As a nation, we chose to add fluoride to our water—not just to the water of people who had cavities. We routinely add iron and other supplements to flour (and, hence, all baked goods). Our enormously expensive antismoking campaign is an example of targeting everyone in the hope of helping a smaller group; after all, not everyone smokes, and not everyone who smokes dies of lung cancer or suffers a heart attack. Should we mandate the public health heart program? Of course not. I'm not suggesting we pump aspirin and statins into public water supplies, but I do think we should seriously consider reclassifying statins as a dietary supplement, so that they would be widely available without a prescription. Some pharmaceutical companies oppose this idea because they have a proprietary interest in keeping their drug prices high. Other, more enlightened companies support the concept if only because they see the potential for billions in profits. Just as they forecasted gloom and doom when ibuprofen (Motrin) became an over-the-counter drug, many doctors, and some in the pharmaceutical industry, are predicting cataclysmic destruction of all we hold dear if statins are sold without a prescription. They were wrong about ibuprofen, and they're wrong about statins. These drugs are safe, and this program will be at the forefront of a sea change in the way we deal with heart disease.

In my practice I see doctors who strut about the hospital, dragging people back from death's door; doing transplants, bypass surgery, cardiac catheterizations, and thinking that they're God's gift to humanity. But there is a group of doctors I know pretty well who treat patients before they reach this point. They're superb physicians—internists and public health doctors, mostly—and even though they don't make as much money as the superstar cardiologists and cardiac surgeons, they go home content with the knowledge that they have saved lives in their own way. And then there are those whose impact is even less obvious, at least to the casual observer: engineers, scientists, activists, doctors—all toiling earnestly, and often in obscurity, to improve public health. This last group may have the greatest impact of all. I see this book as a public health effort as well. With any luck, we're going to broadcast the truth to America and save lives. We'll help people *before* they get sick. And maybe, along the way, we can shut down a few open heart surgery operating rooms and empty a few intensive care units.

I am most impressed by people who are trying to be that oldest brother in the parable, the one who wants to stop disease by preventing its cause; the one who believes, as the Taoist would say, that the best war is that which is never fought. Personally, I am tired of the medical powers that be, the "thought leaders" (an awful phrase, which, by the way, reminds me of George Orwell and *1984*), sitting on information that the American people have enough intelligence to understand, until they, the doctors, decide it's correct and conservatively implementable, until the last *i* is dotted and the last *t* is crossed. I understand hesitation when you're dealing with something that is extremely dangerous or something that has tremendous negative implications for the health of America, something that, if done wrong, will kill people. But I'm talking about information that people have a right to know. Furthermore, if the information looks good, and the risk of using that information is low, and the potential benefit is very high, then withholding the information could condemn a generation to unnecessary premature death. And I'm sick of that! I've seen it too many times before, and that is one of the reasons I've written this book.

You will hear me campaign on these pages for greater and easier access to statins, something generally favored by insurance companies (cynics will say that this is because insurance companies often don't reimburse customers for over-the-counter medications) but opposed by many of my colleagues in the medical community. Physicians are typically conservative people who don't want anything available over the counter, because if you list the side effects of every drug that you have ever taken, you shouldn't be alive. Everything will kill you. I can probably give you enough lettuce to drive you into an early grave. There are those doctors worried about any drug taken by anybody at any time, without close medical supervision. It's a control issue, really, because the process sends you back to the doctor's office; it sends you back for checkups and more observation and more evaluation and less control over your own body. Is it fair to suggest that there is a cabal of doctors? I don't think it's that malevolent or that obvious. More likely, it stems from an attempt, albeit misguided and misinformed, to do the right thing. Every doctor has heard stories about some patient who used too much of some over-the-counter medication and wound up sick. These stories scare the hell out of them. But the doctors don't hear the stories about the 100,000 other people who took these drugs and never showed up at their doorstep at all, because everything was fine. I run an intensive care unit, and I can tell you what I hate: I hate heart surgery, lung surgery, bowel surgery, and vascular surgery. Why? Because some of the people who endure these procedures check into my unit to die. I don't see the thousands of people who go home and get better. It's all a matter of perspective.

I think if you are an intelligent person, then you have a right to interpret the data in this book for yourself. I think that's a reasonable position to take. I can tell you that the government's imposing itself in this situation is another issue that makes many doctors, and many groups dedicated to patients' rights, extremely uncomfortable. If you are subject to death from a disease process, and you know of a therapy that you are willing to try, though you are aware of its risks, the government is still often going to tell you that you can't do it. If you need proof of this, look no further than the acquired immunodeficiency syndrome (AIDS) epidemic, in which there were plenty of people with a death sentence. They knew they had the human immunodeficiency virus (HIV-positive). They knew there were therapies out there that were extraordinarily dangerous and experimental, and they were, of course, willing to try them, with informed consent; yet the federal government wouldn't let them. The FDA was taken to the mat on this one, and the patients' rights advocates, to a large degree, emerged victorious. Their efforts compelled the FDA to accelerate its approval process and to reexamine its mission, and that was a wonderful thing.

The more control people have over their own body, the better.

There is an unspoken assumption in the medical community that your body, your physiological processes, your medication, are *mine*—that is, your doctor's. That's just wrong. In point of fact, doctors only get your body on loan, and only so long as you agree to lend it to them for therapy. If you're an ethical physician you don't do things to people without their consent, and you don't *withhold* things from people without their consent, because the two acts—doing and withholding—in my mind are ethically inseparable. To me, the availability of information that allows a patient to assess his or her risk and then decide whether or not to institute therapy is ethically mandated. Clearly, I'm not going to give someone a lethal poison, such as a chemotherapy agent, to inject at home between lunch and dinner, but I'm not talking about that here. I'm talking about a different view of heart disease, a different model, and empowering people to take care of it on their own. If you don't believe me, and you don't like it, fine. I'm not going to be angry. It's your choice. But I want you to have the information to make that choice.

I'll tell you a story, specifically on point. In the early 1990s I anchored a nightly broadcast on CNBC called *America's Vital Signs*. It was an hour of live health television. One of my guests was Dr. Linus Pauling. There are very few people I've met who simply cause me to sit down and go, *Wow!* Linus Pauling was such a man—brilliant, ethical, a sparkling conversationalist, a genuinely charming guy who even in his late eighties remained sharp and vital and completely without pretense. At the time, Dr. Pauling was known as Dr. Vitamin C, because he was traveling the country proposing that vitamin C not only was the answer to the common cold, but might also be the answer to other diseases, including heart disease and cancer. He was advocating megadoses of vitamin C. Not surprisingly, since Dr. Pauling was not a physician (he was a chemist), the reaction among the medical community was outrage: *How dare he say these things that will influence patients' behavior? He's not an M.D.!* So there we were, live on television, coast to coast, when I said to Dr. Pauling, "You know, doctors don't like you. They object to what you're doing. What do you have to say for yourself?"

He looked at me and he smiled, and he said, "Well, I know doctors don't like me, but that's because I'm paid to think and they're not." I said, "What do you mean?! That's just going to make them angrier."

And then Dr. Pauling offered a fascinating explanation, one that I've never forgotten:

> Most doctors are very intelligent people who execute care plans, which are really cookbooks—lists of things to do for given problems. Doctors are not paid to inquire into root causes, although the good ones do. Most are paid to see patients, interpret what they see, and then correlate that with their list of things to do for these diseases. What I do is different. I ask questions the doctors are not asking, such as, *Why not vitamin C?* There are reasons to believe it works, so why not try it? Doctors get annoyed at me because I'm outside the box. They should instead say, *Let's wait and see what Pauling has found out. Maybe we can use it.*

In fact, Dr. Pauling was philosophically correct, although the jury is still out on vitamin C. In the case of heart disease, it's the same. Doctors are very conservative. They live by the lists of symptoms that correlate to accepted therapies. They don't want to rock the boat; they don't want to suggest something that might harm you, even if the chance of harm is small compared to the possibility that it might help you.

I'm not Linus Pauling, but I don't mind rocking the boat a little either. If my mission as a doctor is to comfort the afflicted, then my mission as a journalist, at least in part, is to afflict the comfortable. That's one of the things I loved about live network television: You could agitate a pompous guest and he couldn't do anything about it but answer your questions.

And it isn't just the snake-oil salesman who can't stand to be challenged. It's often true that the more esteemed the physician, the more likely he is to be offended by any sort of questioning of his authority and expertise. For example, Dr. C. Everett Koop, the former surgeon general of the United States, also appeared on our CNBC show. At that time Dr. Koop was a highly regarded father figure trying to use his position as the former chief doctor of America to promote a political position. In short, he was advocating legislation that would have permitted a dramatic increase in the random, unannounced drug testing of corporate employees, especially those deemed "critical." In preparing for this interview, I spent some time with the in-house attorneys at CNBC, and together we devised a list of questions we considered to be not only important, but fair, for example, a request for an explanation of the word *critical*. Which employees would fall under this umbrella, and why? It seemed a reasonable line of questioning to me, but as the interview went on, it became apparent that Dr. Koop was not happy. Indeed, when we broke for a commercial, I heard he had one of his assistants place a direct call to the news director of CNBC to complain about the aggressive nature of the interview (I never could confirm the phone call, but the looks I got from management for days thereafter spoke volumes).

Doctors, as a group, do not like to be asked "Why?" For two reasons: (1) They don't like having their authority challenged, and (2) they often don't know the answer. "Why?" is a very difficult question, and many doctors don't like to get difficult questions, at least not in public. They've gone through the system and feel they've earned the right to a certain level of respect and authority. You've seen the T-shirts that say "Because I'm the mommy, that's why." Well, that used to be true of doctors, too. But not anymore. That attitude won't cut it in the twenty-first century, not when so many people have access to so much information, people who understand that they have a right to inquire and prod and question, especially about matters that are important to them, such as life and death.

If I sound passionate about this subject, well, it's only because I am. The way we're going to beat heart disease in this country is by informing people that they have options they may not have considered in the past. That's why I consider *The Heart of the Matter* to be a public health book, a book everyone can read and discuss, including the so-called thought leaders and politicians. Will some people be saying, "This guy is full of garbage"? No doubt. But not the smart ones, I hope. Not the scientists and research experts, and certainly not the average person on the street who wants a crack at living a longer, healthier life. A few people will get side effects and stop the treatment. A few will never start. But the rest of us? Ahhh! The rest of us will be dancing on their graves.

If enough people embrace this formula, ours may well be the last generation on Earth to see people die of premature heart disease. A generation from now, in the second half of the twenty-first century, people will be saying, incredulously, "You know, there was a time when it wasn't unusual to die of heart disease at the age of sixty, and not like we do now, at the age of ninety." Wouldn't that be a kick? Better yet, wouldn't it be a kick to be there and see it happen?

CHAPTER TWO

A History Lesson

Thirty years ago, when I was in medical school, heart disease was heart disease. There was angina, which was heart pain, and there was heart attack, which was a sudden cataclysmic disaster during which patients died. In the latter part of the twentieth century this was all presented to us as one disease. The presumption was that you started off getting a little sick, and you had this pain called angina, and then you got a little sicker and the angina happened more often, and then you got *really* sick, and pretty soon you had what was called *crescendo angina* or *unstable angina*, which meant you had heart pain all the time. Typically, when you reached that point, the sirens went off and they rushed you to the hospital, and they bypassed your coronary arteries to get blood to your heart, and then your life was saved and your surgeons were heroes and everyone was happy.

Quite honestly, the central mechanism of all this seemed to make sense at the time (except, of course, for the surgical ego part). The heart, as any organ in the body does, needs oxygen to live. And oxygen is carried to the heart by blood vessels. Granted, it may sound odd that the heart—which of course is a pump that is completely filled with blood and is the motor that pumps blood to every other organ—should ever be in need of blood, but the heart has arteries that carry blood to it, just as any other organ does. It can't live on the blood that's inside the pumping chamber; it lives on the blood that's carried to it by the feeding arteries, the coronary arteries. So, thirty years ago, when the heart had pain, angina, the thinking was, *Ahhh, these coronary arteries are the problem.* When doctors and scientists looked at the arteries of people who experienced this type of heart pain, they found precisely what they were looking for: obstruction in the arteries. When doctors analyzed these obstructions, they found cholesterol and calcium, and the deposits were as hard as rock; in people with more heart pain, there was more obstruction, and in people with less pain, there was less obstruction. All in all, it made sense.

Although the analytical tools we had when I was a student may seem somewhat primitive by today's standards, they were practically the stuff of science fiction when compared with those available to physicians working in the latter part of the nineteenth century. It's interesting to read the medical literature from a century ago. Doctors knew back then that people had heart disease and that they often died from it. They also knew there wasn't a lot they could do for them. Yes, there were a few drugs—so-called heart tonics, such as nitroglycerin and digitalis—that affected patients in some way, and so they presumed that the drugs were useful. These drugs could ease the discomfort of heart disease, but they couldn't prevent the disease from getting worse over time. If you were unfortunate enough to be a victim of heart disease in the latter part of the nineteenth century, when you started feeling this pain, the clock started ticking. We had no technology to do anything for you. You had no choice but to hope for the best and wait for the day when your illness might contribute to the greater good, in the form of a postmortem exam.

We had the technology to examine the effects of heart disease—after the fact—and we learned a lot from these exams. The old name for heart attack was *coronary thrombosis*, which means, literally, a clot in the coronary arteries. Doctors saw blood clots in the coronary arteries of people who had died of heart attacks. The doctors presumed that the clots had caused the attacks. Later doctors pooh-poohed this idea and backed away from it. We know today that the old theory was correct: that a clot in the coronary artery *is* the cause of heart attack. Furthermore, if you actually go back through history, you'll find evidence that a great many doctors and scientists were sniffing around the edges of other such discoveries. Consider this statement from an article titled "The relationship between acute infectious disease and arterial lesions" in the *Archives of Internal Medicine*: "The sclerosis of old age may simply be a summation of lesions arising from infections or metabolic toxins." In other words, maybe this heart disease stems from infection. Interesting, considering not only that it's probably true, but that this article was published in 1911!

The very limitations of technology around the turn of the twentieth century may have prompted some progressive, even daring thinking. This was the age of the great observational doctors, who worked at a time when it wasn't possible to examine the living, beating heart of a human being. Bypass surgery, coronary ultrasound, catheterization—these were tools no one had even dreamed of inventing. All a doctor could do was look at his patients, talk to them, listen to them. Maybe that wasn't such a bad thing, because the observational doctors developed extraordinary diagnostic skills. There were, however, limitations to what their eyes, ears, and fingers could tell them about what was wrong with an organ buried deep in the chest and beating ceaselessly an average of seventy times a minute. In the end, it always seemed to come down to this: bad heart, cause unknown. Whatever the reason, the heart simply gave out, and even if these doctors knew the reason—even if they knew for certain that there was a link between heart disease and infectious disease, for example—there was nothing they could do, because there were no antibiotics available until the middle of the twentieth century.

So we had all these brilliant physicians wondering whether infection could cause heart disease, noticing that there were blood clots in coronary arteries, calling the condition by its name—*coronary thrombosis*—and yet being unable to do anything about it. It must have been a terribly frustrating time for them. They were powerless to affect anything. The scientific method was just starting to come into its own in medicine; you could ask some basic questions and then you could expect answers. The first obvious question was, *What causes this?* That would prompt scientific study, which would end with an answer, *Now I know.* The next obvious question would be, *How can we stop it?* For infectious disease, the answer was in the form of antibiotics almost halfway through the twentieth century. For heart disease the answer has been much slower in coming.

Doctors typically lumped all heart disease together. Angina pain, heart attack—they were all pieces of the same puzzle, or so it was thought. Conditions changed subtly with the advent of the heart-lung bypass machine, which made it possible to "bypass" damaged coronary arteries, arteries clogged with plaque or debris. New arteries were fashioned out of pieces of vein taken from elsewhere in a patient's body and then plugged into the heart to keep the blood flowing freely to feed heart muscle tissue. The coronary artery bypass graft (CABG) operation was popularized in the late 1960s and soon became routine. By the 1980s, it was the most commonly performed major surgery in the United States. Why? Because heart disease was (and still is) the leading killer in America, and we thought we finally had a tool to fight it effectively. The coronary artery bypass graft was considered, at first, revolutionary. It was also, in the early days, extraordinarily dangerous. You wouldn't bypass arteries unless you had sufficient evidence that there was a problem in them. How did we get this evidence? Through the use of a coronary angiogram (first demonstrated in 1959), which was a sophisticated X ray of the coronary arteries. It showed the lumps and bumps of plaque bulging into and obstructing the flow of coronary artery blood.

With the angiogram we could observe, for the first time, exactly what was happening in the living human heart, and what we observed was that there was a lot of trouble in there. It confirmed what we thought we knew from the autopsies performed on people who had died of heart attacks.

Autopsy suites often have a version of the famous phrase "From the dead to help the living" posted somewhere prominently. I observed as many autopsies as possible at Columbia Presbyterian Hospital during my first year in medical school because I quickly learned that an autopsy provided the best educational bang for your buck. "The Man in the Pan" (an awful phrase, I know, but that's what we called it) was a brilliant teacher. Every morning, the pathologist would present the major findings of all the autopsies done the previous day. There would be a pan brimming with organs—the heart, the liver, the spleen—and I thought they were so dramatic, and so critical to understanding why disease does what it does that I got up at six in the morning every day to attend. The most dramatic moment I remember was the first time I watched the pathologist display the heart of someone who had died of a heart attack. He showed us this heart, wide open, with nothing obviously wrong. Then he opened the coronary arteries, and he took a small metallic pick and ran it along the inside of the artery, and you could hear a little noise: *tink-tink-tink*, as if he was hitting something hard—the same awful noise you hear in your head when the dentist is scraping at your teeth.

"You see this?" the pathologist said. "This is plaque."

"What's plaque?" I wondered aloud.

"Well, Salgo, if you'd been listening to the lectures, you'd know. It's a piece of calcified rock."

It was amazing to me that this horrible stuff actually grew inside the arteries feeding the human heart. You didn't have to be a rocket scientist to know that having plaque in your arteries was a bad thing. If left untreated, I learned, the plaque grew larger, until it choked off the blood supply. In people who died of heart attacks, plaque almost completely obstructed the arteries; the heart attack was often associated with a blood clot right at the site of the plaque. This was all new to me, even though it had been fairly common knowledge for decades that plaque caused problems. Autopsies, after all, had been part and parcel of medical science for some time, and in the normal course of an autopsy, a doctor would cut open a coronary artery, find some plaque, and quickly make the determination that plaque had obstructed the flow of blood through the artery. Blood feeds the heart, of course, so if the plaque continues to grow, eventually it can cause a heart attack. All of this was told to me when I was a medical student (as it's told to every medical student), and my reaction was, "Sounds reasonable."

As with most doctors in the 1970s, I didn't give it much more thought. *Prevent the plaque* was the mantra of the day. Prevent plaque from forming and you prevent heart attacks: simple as that. And the angiogram, a wonderful invention, allowed us to find evidence of plaque in patients who were not yet dead. All you had to do was inject a little dye into the coronary arteries and watch the dye flow. A funny thing, too: When you look at an angiogram, you look at where the dye isn't. In other words, if the pipe leading to the heart, carrying blood, is wide open, there will be blood everywhere. The dye, which looks white on the X-ray tube, fills the artery smoothly from wall to wall. But if there's a piece of plaque stuck to the artery wall, you'll see a big black hole, because the flow of blood is obstructed by the plaque.

The simple angiogram not only paved the way for bypass surgery, it led directly to angioplasty, too. Angioplasty is a procedure in which a thin balloon is introduced through an artery, usually in the groin, and snaked up the major conduit of blood, the aorta, that leads to the heart. From there, it's slipped into a coronary artery and positioned over one of those "black holes," presumably the plaque stuck to the arterial wall. Then the balloon is inflated and the plaque crushed. If everything works as it should, normal, smooth blood flow is restored and all becomes right with the world. The basic premise is the same for both bypass surgery and angioplasty: Where there is obstruction to flow, there's hard, calcified plaque sticking into the artery and clogging up the works. And plaque is dangerous. It can lead to heart attacks.

All of this seemed great and useful and explained a lot. But there were a few points it didn't explain. For example, every doctor, me included, has seen patients such as Mr. Jones. Mr. Jones is about fifty years old, and he calls the office and says: "Gee, Doc, everything was fine. I've been playing tennis all my life, and I've been running, and—I don't know. I just got home from work and I've got this really nasty pain in my chest, and it's kind of dull and persistent and squeezy, and it feels like there's an elephant on my chest. It's radiating down my left arm into my jaw, into my neck; I'm a little short of breath; and I'm sweating and it's getting worse, and I've got to tell you, I feel like crap."

Any doctor worth his diploma will hear that description and immediately say, "Come into the hospital, you're having a heart attack." But the strange thing about our Mr. Jones is that he didn't have any previous symptoms. How do we explain that? If the heart attack is caused by the slow steady progression of calcified plaque to the point that it gradually obstructs a coronary artery, then this guy doesn't fit the model at all. And if he doesn't fit the model, then suddenly the model doesn't make sense. Where is the classic description, "My heart pain started twenty years ago, and it got worse year by year. Then suddenly I couldn't climb the stairs, and then I couldn't get out of a chair. Then I came to the hospital"? Typically, after this long and agonizing process of obstruction, the guy would have a heart attack and then bypass surgery, and the cycle would start all over again. But not Mr. Jones. Where did his heart attack come from? Well, we didn't know. But we did know this: There were a lot of people like Mr. Jones. In fact, close to 50 percent of heart attack victims fit his profile, and it was a mystifying profile indeed.

On patients such as Mr. Jones, we usually did an angiogram, and we usually saw obstruction to flow, and we often presumed there was some type of blood clot in the artery. Often these patients did have plaque, but we couldn't be sure whether that plaque was large enough to cause the symptoms we were seeing. Left with few options, we usually bypassed these patients or angioplastied them, with good results. That may sound a bit disconcerting—the notion that surgery, even successful surgery, was performed without rock-solid (no pun intended) evidence that it was the proper course of action—but it must be considered in the proper historical context. We all thought that heart disease was the slow, steady progression of plaque, obstructing the coronary arteries until the point where the heart couldn't live anymore. I think mechanically. Surgeons do and cardiologists, too. In a way, doctors, especially doctors who specialize in cardiac care, are really just plumbers: *Uh-oh, the pipes are rusty. Better bypass the rust!* And that's what we did. There was always a lot of rust and calcified gunk in there, so we'd reroute the blood around the obstruction or crush the obstruction out of the way. Conceptually it's no more complicated than building an alternative pathway around the beaver dam, so that you can drain the pond and keep water flowing downstream.

The beauty of this procedure lies in its simplicity and elegance. Coronary artery bypass grafting does make sense in a lot of ways. If you see an obstructed coronary artery, there has to be some fallout—typically, a heart that needs oxygen. So you go in and bypass the coronary artery and save a life and everyone goes home happy. The procedure has improved greatly in recent years, to the point that it is now possible to have so-called minimally invasive bypass surgery and not even go on the bypass pump. But it's still major surgery. Everyone who endures bypass surgery goes directly to the intensive care unit postoperatively. All of them get powerful drugs. There are all kinds of consequences to this surgery that are unexpected. For the longest time, though, it was the only option. There is an old medical phrase: Desperate diseases require desperate measures. The early bypass surgeries were desperate measures. Doctors (and patients) were involved in a race against the obstruction, the implacable enemy was death, and the risk worth taking was almost anything. The point is this: The risk of the surgery was death.

But the risk of no operation was death, too. So the only question, it seemed, was which was more likely to kill you, the surgery or the heart disease.

Surgery had other risks, too. Stroke was one; infection was another. So if a person just survived the surgery, that wasn't enough to recommend the procedure. The patient had to come out the other side of the operating room experience both alive and intact for the operation to be considered worthwhile.

But wait a minute. You could "stroke out" after a heart attack, too. And a heart attack could leave you with so much dead heart tissue that what was left pumping was barely adequate to get you out of bed to the bathroom each day. That was a terrible "nondeath" outcome, too. The decision to operate always involved a balancing act. We all spent a lot of time comparing the risks of operating with those of waiting.

And so the big debate centered around whether the surgery was really significantly better than conservative medical management. Doctors had newer, better heart drugs every year: beta-blockers, calcium channel blockers, and the like. All of these were drugs that decreased the heart's need for oxygen. This reduced demand would make the heart happier with the reduced supply it was getting from its plaque-clogged arteries. But you never get something for nothing. These drugs decreased the heart's need for oxygen by decreasing its pumping power. Think of it this way: You can decrease your car's gas requirement by removing two of its cylinders. You'll get better mileage, but you're not going to get anywhere very fast. It's a trade-off.

Over the years the evidence seemed to support the notion that, in the short term, surgery was a pretty dangerous choice. You were more likely to die of the operation than you were of another heart attack in the next few years. But it wasn't quite that simple, for the evidence also demonstrated that if you survived the initial operation and emerged stroke-free, there were significant benefits down the line. Successful bypass surgery not only seemed to extend your life (statistically at least), but improved the quality of your life by eradicating the pain of angina. And if angina was the screaming complaint of a heart in desperate need of oxygen, then the mechanism of bypass surgery to provide more blood to the heart made perfect sense.

But there remained a nagging issue, which, because we couldn't do much to resolve it, most people ignored, and that was this: Bypass surgery sure as hell was a great way to relieve angina, but it wasn't nearly as good at keeping you alive longer. Sure, if you had massive heart disease, triple-vessel disease, three, four coronary arteries involved, bypass surgery not only relieved your angina, it saved your life. If you had one or two coronary arteries involved, though, it would relieve your angina but didn't necessarily do anything to prolong your life. That was perplexing. Why wasn't this always a dramatic lifesaving procedure? Why didn't it always have a dramatic, almost binary effect: *You're going to die if you don't have it; you won't die if you do?* That is the question that has been nagging at cardiologists, internists, and surgeons for a great many years.

At least, I know it's been nagging at me.

I had a unique case about five years ago. I was on duty in the ICU, in the middle of the night, when a gentleman arrived in great distress. He was perhaps sixty years old and clearly having a heart attack. No question about it. In addition to crushing pain in his chest, this man had the electrocardiographic evidence of a heart attack—specific changes in his cardiogram—as well as falling blood pressure and a dangerously irregular heart rhythm. These are all conditions a heart attack causes just before it kills you. There was no doubt that this man had to go straight down to the cardiac catheterization lab and have his

coronary arteries examined. If we found a problem we were going to bypass or angioplasty him. So we hooked him up to all the
modern technology at our disposal, ran a catheter into his groin,
injected some dye into his coronary artery, took a picture, and
predictably saw an obstructed artery. No surprise. What happened next, however, was a surprise. After we injected a little
more dye, lo and behold, something moved, and suddenly the
coronary artery reopened, and the heart attack ended—just like
that. The presumption among those of us in the room was that
we had seen a coronary blood clot: the old "coronary thrombosis" rearing its ugly head again. Not hard, calcified plaque, but
a big, gelatinous blob that for some reason just slithered out of
the way. We had flushed the clot out with only a little squirt of
dye. As I watched it move, I thought to myself, *Hmmmm, isn't
that interesting*. The patient, naturally, didn't care what had
happened, only that he instantly felt better. Within a few days he
was discharged.

I hadn't seen anything like it before. Most of the cardiologists
had, but I hadn't, and frankly I found it shocking. I'd been taking care of this man in the ICU, and he'd been so sick that he
needed me to go with him to the cath lab. It never occurred to
me that he was suffering from something that could be fixed—
accidentally or intentionally—quite so quickly. Where was his
hard plaque? He didn't have any. Where was the balloon
catheter to crush the offending calcium? We didn't need it.

The cardiologists had become inured to this phenomenon,
but I couldn't help wondering, *Where is this clot really coming
from, and how can we prevent it from coming back?* There was
something strange going on, something I didn't completely understand. I hoped that the cardiologists understood it, but in
point of fact they didn't really understand it either. No one did.
Everybody just sort of whistled past the graveyard, clinging to

the assumption that heart disease was heart disease, plaque was plaque, and eventually, if you accumulated enough plaque, you were going to have a heart attack, so we needed to treat plaque.

But there were other niggling issues in all of this. For example, lots of diet doctors claimed that if you ate a low-cholesterol diet, your heart attack risk would go down. But down from what? Down from the national average, or down from the risk with your particular heart—your particular physiological, chemical, and genetic makeup? In other words, would a low-cholesterol diet make that plaque go away? I never understood why, if you ate a low-cholesterol diet, calcium would be absorbed into your body and disappear somehow. In fact, there was substantial evidence to show that *didn't* happen. Hard plaque was there, and it stuck. Maybe, through diet and exercise, you could prevent the accumulation of more hard plaque, but you certainly weren't going to make the stuff that was already there go away. Lots of us read the diet claims and scoffed. But there was some evidence that the diets worked; they reduced your heart attack risk. So some of us wondered whether the diet results were telling us something about heart attack we didn't yet understand. If the hard plaque didn't go away, yet your heart attack risk decreased, went the argument, did that imply that something other than hard plaque was causing heart attacks?

Cholesterol is an important issue, and we'll address it in great length, but here's a preliminary word about it. People assume that we know why heart disease occurs: If you eat too much cholesterol, you're going to get heart disease. If you ask your average cardiologist, he'll say, "Yes, your lipid profile, the amount of fat and the kind of fat in your blood, *is* very important." And he's right about that. Your lipid profile *is* very important; the accumulation of cholesterol does cause heart attacks.

But that doesn't answer the question Why? It answers the question What? Furthermore, there are other factors, aside from cholesterol, that are associated with heart attack: high blood pressure, for example; weight; smoking. There's a whole list of things that contribute to heart disease, and although we know there is a demonstrated statistical correlation, that doesn't necessarily tell us why they exist.

There were several landmark epidemiology studies done in the middle of the twentieth century, the most famous of which was the Framingham Study, in Framingham, Massachusetts. An absolutely remarkable, groundbreaking effort, the Framingham Study took an entire town's population and examined it in astounding detail. The researchers obtained mind-numbingly intricate records of the participants' lives: what they ate, how much they weighed, what their blood pressure was, how much they exercised, whether or not they smoked. Then the researchers sat back and watched as these people lived their lives. The epidemiologists kept records and calculated death rates, sickness rates, and so on, and from Framingham we learned that cholesterol was indeed an extremely important issue. So were weight, smoking, blood pressure, and a host of other factors. There were other studies, too, but Framingham is widely regarded, even today, as the gold standard. From Framingham originated the doctor's mantra: *Change your diet! Exercise more! Throw away your cigarettes!* Some of that, especially the last item, may sound like common sense today, but remember, as recently as the late 1940s, not only were cigarettes not deemed to be a risk, but there were advertisements in the mainstream media that boasted of the health benefits of smoking. I have one of them on a wall in my office, an almost Rockwellian depiction of a doctor strolling happily past a picket fence and into someone's home, black bag in tow, a cigarette dangling from his lip. The implication was that if you smoked the doctor's brand of cigarette, you were in good shape.

That all changed with Framingham. There's nothing like epidemiology to put the nail in a risk-factor's coffin. Framingham told us, in no uncertain terms, that smoking was bad. We didn't know exactly what it did that caused harm, but we sure as hell knew that if you smoked you were a lot more likely to die than if you didn't smoke. We didn't know why, because epidemiology is not designed to tell you why; it tells you what. That's a critical distinction, one the public often misperceives. They think doctors and scientists know why smokers die of heart disease. Well, we didn't then, and we don't know for certain even now (though we'll explore a tantalizing clue in the infectious disease chapter). I mean, we know that if you smoke a cigarette, the carbon monoxide level in your blood goes up, because anything that burns produces carbon monoxide. We know that the carbon monoxide attaches to hemoglobin, which is the molecule in the blood that carries oxygen to the tissues, and that the hemoglobin molecule is then unavailable to carry oxygen. Therefore, we know that the amount of oxygen delivered to the tissues decreases and the heart becomes starved for oxygen. That's a very bad thing, but it still doesn't explain precisely *why* smoking makes you die of a heart attack. For one thing, the lack of oxygen should produce terrible damage immediately. If I took a drag on a cigarette, and then I clutched my chest and keeled over dead, maybe that would help explain why smoking kills. But it usually doesn't work that way. Smoking cigarettes produces a cumulative risk that adds up over time and persists long after a smoker has quit. If you ask me to tell you, molecule by molecule, what it is about cigarette smoke that kills you, or makes you predisposed to a heart attack, even when you're not smoking a cigarette—and people do die of heart attacks five years after they quit—I can't. And I'll tell you something else: neither can anyone else. Am I picking nits? I don't think so. Why are you still sick five years down the line? Did you knock off heart cells along the way? Probably not, but nobody knows for sure.

It's a wonderful thing to know *why* as well as *what*. For example, if I have pneumococcal pneumonia, I know there's a pneumococcus bacterium having lunch in my lung. I know why I'm sick. I know if I get a dose of penicillin, the pneumococcus goes away and I get better. I have a cause, I have an effect, I have a therapy based on the cause. What does all this have to do with heart disease? Simple: I'm telling you that cardiology, unlike infectious disease and until the new information we'll be examining in this book became available, was based almost entirely on observational, epidemiologic data rather than root cause data. That is to say, only now do we know why some of the well-known risk factors described by the Framingham researchers increase your risk of dying of a coronary thrombosis. The Framingham Study found powerful statistical associations between cigarettes, hypertension, high cholesterol level, overweight, and lack of exercise and heart disease. You can't do that in a small study. You need thousands of people observed over decades. That's what makes Framingham so remarkable, so brilliant.

After Framingham began to publish its results (and it is still publishing, still studying), we knew what affected your heart disease risk, but not how many of these risk factors caused damage. We knew how you should live, what to avoid, what factors contributed to and were associated with living longer, but we didn't know why. If you really wanted to confuse a cardiologist in the 1970s, all you had to say was, "I've got all the manuals; I've got all the books; I've stopped smoking, changed my diet; I exercise more; I've lost weight. Now, tell me why I'm doing this."

"Why, to live longer, of course," the cardiologist would say.

At that point either you could walk out of the office, content in the knowledge that you were doing the right thing, even if you didn't understand why, or you could drive the cardiologist mad by asking a simple follow-up question:

"Yeah, but why? Why will it make me live longer?"

In response, the doctor would most likely give you his best wide-eyed impersonation of Ralph Kramden: "Hamana-hamana-hamana."

Translation: "I don't know."

I always found it intriguing that heart disease had two flavors. One was the slow, progressive heart pain we called *angina*, described through history, in all common literature, as a squeezing heart pain that predictably got worse over time and that we could treat with medicine. The other flavor was far more sudden and cataclysmic: heart *attack*. People who suffered heart attacks were dying right then! Chronic medication that took years to work wasn't going to help them during their minutes or hours of peril. It always seemed to me that there was a distinction between these two types of heart disease, angina and heart attack, and yet this distinction was not being examined effectively enough for me in the literature, or in what I had been taught as a medical student and as a young doctor. When I saw someone gravely ill with a heart attack, I couldn't help but wonder, *What's wrong with the picture I was taught?* Especially since I would often see people who had experienced no angina, no symptoms, none of what you expected to see in someone who is terribly ill with heart disease, but were dying of heart attack nonetheless. I'd see someone who walked into the emergency room and said: "I ran a marathon three weeks ago, and now I have crushing heart pain. What's happening to me?" I didn't have the answer. Well, I sort of had the answer—"You're having a heart attack!"—but I didn't have an explanation. So I wondered what it was I had not been taught. Here we were, in the latter part of the twentieth century, presumably with every technological miracle at our disposal, bypassing people left and right, performing catheterizations and angioplasty on an hourly basis, using every tool known to medical science to make a proper and educated diagnosis, and still something was missing. If the explanation that I had been taught in medical school was correct—that heart disease was a gradual process, with bypass or death due to heart attack the end point—then this poor guy sitting in front of me, the one who had run the marathon, simply shouldn't be in my office.

But there he was.

You know, the human body is a classic example of what I like to call Murphy's law of biology: "Under the most carefully controlled conditions of temperature, pressure, and humidity, the organism does what it damn well pleases." It's not like theoretical physics. I was trained as a physicist in college, and in physics matters are really clean. You say to yourself: "I've got a presumptive mechanism for the way stars shine, and if they're shining this way by fusing hydrogen into helium, then I should see these characteristics. I'll just do a spectrographic analysis through my telescope, and *bada-bing!* there it is. Look at that! I'm a genius!" Biology is the other way around. It's much more of an empirical science, an observational science. You don't ask "Why?" first. You ask, "What's going on here?" You set up a Framingham Study. You observe, and then, later, you try to find an explanation that fits your observations. It's the opposite of theoretical physics, and it's much more complicated and intuitive. In fact, the more you look at the human body, the more you realize that it is hideously complicated, and that for every simple, straightforward, clean-cut explanation, there is some patient who will come along and prove to you that you are an absolute idiot.

The more I hung around and observed, the more I saw patients like the marathon man—patients who didn't fit the profile of slow, intrusive, irreversible plaque building up in the coronary artery, squeezing the life out of the artery, much as a boa constrictor squeezes the life out of its victim. They were feeling fine one day and having a catastrophic blow the next. (It's interesting, too, isn't it, the nomenclature we give these things? It tells us something if we're willing to listen. *Angina pectoris* simply means "chest pain," whereas *heart attack* has the word *attack* in it. *Attack* implies something much more aggressive and unexpected: a disaster. They sound like two different things, and in fact they are quite different. If we had been sensitive to the syntax, we'd have pricked up our ears much earlier.) The presumption was that a heart attack was the final stage of vascular rusting, that the arteries eventually deteriorated to the point that the heart couldn't breathe anymore, and you died. If that were the case, however, then every patient who suffered a heart attack would have had a history of angina: of pain. Almost invariably, the scenario would have played out in the following fashion: pain during exertion, pain at rest, pain all the time, then unbearable pain, followed by a trip to the hospital and a date with the surgeon's knife. That wasn't the way it worked. Oh, sure, sometimes it did, but there were sufficient deviations from the norm to cause considerable consternation: patients who were just living their life, pain-free, blissfully unaware of any problem at all. Some had even displayed completely normal cardiograms within a month or so of their heart attack. And then— BANG! They'd find themselves in the back of an ambulance, fighting for their life.

Let's look again at the story of Jim Fixx, the noted running guru and author. He died of a heart attack after running how many marathons? After writing how many books about running marathons? Now, if he had experienced progressive angina, there is no way he would have been able to run a 10K, let alone a marathon. So what's wrong with the Jim Fixx picture?

There were other points that made no sense. How could we account for the fact that improved diet and increased exercise worked as a tool in the fight against heart disease? If the calcium and plaque were there to stay, how could diet and exercise make risk go down?

The traditional explanation also failed to address the fact that aspirin prevented second heart attacks. (Incidentally, there is plenty of literature to suggest it prevents first heart attacks, too, but more on that a little later.) The classic explanation was that aspirin is an anticoagulant. Over time, the hard plaque makes your coronary arteries increasingly narrow and thus impedes and slows the flow of blood. Everyone who has ever cut himself knows that when blood pools, it clots, so it wasn't a great leap of science to suggest that aspirin, as an anticoagulant, prevents blood from clotting, and in that way prevents the coronary thrombosis from forming. In other words, it prevents a heart attack.

But they failed to answer an obvious question: How come it works even though aspirin is a pretty weak anticoagulant? You didn't know that? Well, it's true. When was the last time you took an aspirin, cut yourself shaving, and bled to death? Never, right? That's because it doesn't happen. Oh, sure, aspirin has some anticoagulant properties, but it's nothing like warfarin (Coumadin) or heparin, two of the more powerful and popular blood thinners now in use. Cut yourself shaving while on Coumadin and you've got a serious problem; you'll bleed out.

But aspirin? The truth is, it's not very strong. Yes, we take people off aspirin preoperatively, because a lot of blood loss can occur and we want to err on the side of caution, but it would be inaccurate to suggest that aspirin is a wonderful anticoagulant.

Neither did the traditional explanation address the issue of infectious disease and its apparent link to heart disease. In short, there were a lot of holes in the classical theory of heart attack, holes that were widening with each passing year. You could choose to ignore the evidence, of course; you could cling to the stodgy old notion that heart disease is merely an accumulation of rust in the coronary arteries, and nothing more, but you did so at your own risk. To me, and to others, it became clear that heart disease is really two diseases. One is angina, heart pain. We could treat it with nitroglycerin and other medication to reduce the heart's requirement for oxygen; we could treat it with bypass surgery or angioplasty. All of these treatments worked pretty well. But then there was heart *attack*. Nitroglycerin wouldn't prevent a heart attack. Although there was some effect of angioplasty and bypass surgery, it was not as dramatic as it should have been if the mechanism was what we understood it to be. All of this information was speaking to us, saying something worthwhile, but we weren't listening.

CHAPTER THREE

The Lightbulb Goes On

As recently as the early 1990s, heart disease remained largely a mystery, and our efforts to prevent people from dying of heart attacks were only moderately successful. I had spent fifteen years of my medical career taking care of heart patients and wondering about the cause of all this mayhem in my spare time. I didn't have much spare time; no doctor I know in clinical practice does. So I drifted along from day to day without making much progress in my attempt to understand the processes causing the confusing symptoms I was seeing each day.

My original training was as an internist, so I would spend night after night in the coronary care unit, wandering around, talking to patients, holding their hands, wondering how they had come to be in such a dreadful state. That's what you do as an internist—you try to figure out what's harming your patients and help them get better. But it's tough when you don't have a lot to offer. I can't tell you the number of times I saw acute heart attacks in the emergency room. I felt pretty helpless there, too.

I've never had an office practice, mainly because, at an early age, I became hopelessly addicted to the Sturm und Drang of intensive care medicine. It seemed to me that there simply wasn't enough juice in an office setting; it didn't suit my nervous system to monitor a small group of people slowly, over many years. I liked making a difference—quickly. I am well aware of the great good often done by family practitioners and other doctors who work in private practice, and I'm sure it's an immensely rewarding career path. It's just not for me. I knew very early in my medical training that I wanted to work with people in dire trouble and try to make an immediate impact on their lives.

Maybe that's just a long-winded way of saying that I'm an adrenaline junkie, but it happens to be true. A lot of people who go into intensive care medicine are like that. In many ways it's similar to the surgeon's attitude. Surgeons are fond of saying "A chance to cut is a chance to cure." Well, for the intensivist, a chance to get somebody into your ICU—someone who is going to live or die on the basis of the decisions you make—is a chance to make a difference.

I figured all this out during my residency in internal medicine. I was casting about for something fun to do with my career, and I met a remarkable physician, an anesthesiologist named Dr. Henrik Bendixen. Dr. Bendixen was chairman of the Department of Anesthesiology. He was a larger-than-life figure who is widely regarded as the father of the modern ICU. Dr. Bendixen was Danish by birth and had a remarkable history. He was rumored to have been part of the resistance during World War II, served in the Korean War, and then invented much of the technology that led to intensive care medicine. He had an encyclopedic knowledge of art, music, and wine. He was a cosmopolitan world traveler and had directed academic departments across the United States. I didn't know any of this when I was a medical resident. I just looked at my schedule one day and found I had been assigned to a month in the intensive care unit with this anesthesiologist Bendixen. I remember thinking, *My goodness, what could an anesthesiologist possibly teach me about medicine?* The answer, as it turned out, was *everything*. This man was brilliant. He changed my life. After I finished my medical residency, I went to see Dr. Bendixen and asked whether I could climb on board as one of his residents to train in anesthesiology. I wanted to use both of these specialties to practice intensive care medicine. Fortunately for me, Dr. Bendixen agreed, so I did training in anesthesiology next and then began a career as an intensivist.

I've always been focused on acutely ill patients, whether in the operating room or in the ICU. There's really only a shade of difference between the two settings. For years I was on the heart transplant team, doing anesthesia for cases that occurred in the middle of the night. But waiting for the whir of chopper blades at three o'clock in the morning got old, so I gradually moved toward a career exclusively in the ICU, and that's where I am now.

Who can predict where life will take him next? Not I. I didn't know that events were conspiring to put me in exactly the right place, at the right time, with the right training and access to understand what people were finding out about heart disease. All I knew was that I was seeing some terrible stuff. I still do.

Most of my career has been spent mopping up the debris of the heart disease war. I see people at the end of their disease state; I see people whose ability to lead a normal life has been ravaged by this disease; I have seen people in terrible distress, fighting for their lives, despite the fact that just a few weeks earlier they appeared to be in perfectly good health. I've watched, powerless, from the bedside as they got into more trouble. As the years went by I acquired more tools to help these people, but it became increasingly apparent to me that the time to help them was not when they were on a gurney in the emergency room, writhing in pain, short of breath, clutching their chest; the time to help them was *before* any of this happened.

I kept asking the big question: "How do you prevent this from happening?" I finally realized I was not going to find the answer in the ICU or the operating room. The only way to attack this problem was to attack it early in its course. You move these patients, and their care, to the arena of preventive medicine, which lacks panache. After all, the preventive medicine folks are the people who tell you to eat your Wheaties, go out and exercise, lose weight, and quit smoking. For someone wired as an intensive care doc, this stuff looked boring!

But this is precisely the arena in which heart disease belongs, because, as it turns out, if you want to get a handle on heart disease, you want to avoid ever having to see me. From a patient's perspective, boring is good. Or as a lot of docs like to say, "You never, ever want to be an interesting case!" If you see me staring down at you, oh, man, you have done something wrong. Really wrong! When people ask what I do for a living, I typically just shake my head and say, "You don't want to know, because if you need to know what I do for a living, you're in a fight for your life."

So the object of this book is to keep you away from me. There are doctors in other fields who say, "Seeing me is the best thing that could happen to you." You know—for your checkup, your cosmetic surgery, whatever. I'm not like that. By the time you see me, the you-know-what has already hit the fan.

Those of us who work with hearts tend to treat what we see, not what we can't see. To a hammer, everything is a nail; to a cardiologist or an intensivist, all heart disease stems from plaque. Why? Because that's what we see. The angiogram lets us view plaque, not just at postmortem but in life, and suddenly we have the opportunity to jump at these lesions and bypass them or crush them. Unfortunately, the great disappointment of cardiology in the 1970s, 1980s, and 1990s was that although the technology did save lives, it didn't work quite as well as it should have. Something was wrong. Some piece of the puzzle was missing. All of the lifestyle stuff—stop smoking, exercise more, change your diet—was based on the epidemiological features of heart disease. It didn't explain the biological processes of heart disease. Everyone thought that the biological characteristics were key to understanding heart attacks. But the biological features weren't making much sense.

The confusing fog that surrounded the biology began to clear a little about ten years ago. It started with a broadening of the epidemiologic net to include risk factors for heart attack that no one had bothered to take seriously. For example, instead of just looking at diet and exercise (and other lifestyle issues), a few doctors started considering additional factors, including chronic infections. If you're wondering why anyone would look to infectious disease research for a heart attack solution, consider the story of ulcer disease.

A generation ago, everybody "knew" the cause of ulcers: acid. The typical ulcer patient was a high-stress executive who wore a white shirt, red tie, and blue suit to work every day and kept a bottle of Maalox in his desk drawer. He was under enormous pressure, and that's why he had an ulcer. Moreover, he exacerbated the condition with a bad diet. The logic wasn't entirely flawed. We knew, for instance, that if you had an ulcer, and you ate a chili dog, your stomach would hurt afterward. It also hurt when you experienced stress. A very simple equation, right?

Not really. More recently we've discovered the existence of a bacterium known as *Helicobacter pylori*, which is present in a disturbing number of people who have ulcers. For a while the news of the possible link between *H. pylori* and ulcers was restricted to the medical community and even there mentioned only in hushed tones. But in the last ten to fifteen years, it's percolated into the public arena, so deeply, in fact, that today there are many doctors and scientists who are willing to say that virtually every stomach ulcer is due to an infection in the stomach. If you treat the bacterium that causes the infection, *H. pylori*, with antibiotics, the ulcer goes away. If this is true, then suddenly everything we thought we knew about ulcers is subject to revision. The epidemiology was right, but the cause was something we hadn't suspected from the epidemiologic characteristics. Now you can go ahead and have your three-martini lunch (although with the tax structure the way it is, you can't find anyone to pay for it) and not worry that it's the martini that is causing your stomach pain—or the chili dog, or the stress at work. All of these will make your ulcer hurt more, but they're not the cause. The cause is a tiny microorganism.

Predictably, this development led some astute observers to consider infectious disease as a cause for other diseases that we never suspected were infectious in origin, such as rheumatoid arthritis (RA). RA remains a mystery. We say, "Oh, it's an autoimmune problem," as if that explains everything. *Autoimmune* means the body is allergic to itself. That's not much help, really. After all, what started the autoimmune process? Mark my words, the odds are that you'll be reading a decade from now that rheumatoid arthritis is associated with infectious disease.

Not so long ago, it would have been unthinkable to suggest a link between infectious disease and heart attack, but now it doesn't seem so crazy at all.

As people realized that the clean, simple explanation for heart disease wasn't clean at all, a distinction between angina and heart attack became important. Were they the same disease? Were they related in some way? Were they two different diseases, both of which affected the heart? So they began to focus on the differences between these two problems. If angina and heart attack are different processes, and we have been trying to prevent heart attacks with therapy that only works for angina, that might explain some of the failures of what should have been terrific heart attack techniques, namely, angioplasty and bypass surgery. It might also explain why some therapies that shouldn't have worked against heart attack, diet, for example, seemed to provide some benefit.

Then we found out that people who had heart attacks were more likely than others to have chronic infectious disease. Numerous types of infections were mentioned, but the one that kept cropping up was chlamydia pneumonia. Nobody in the modern era had thought in terms of infectious disease as a cause of heart attack, just as nobody had thought in terms of infectious disease for ulcers. What did these diseases have in common? Typically, they were surgically treated. *A hole in your stomach? A rock in your coronary artery? How could they possibly be due to a bacterium? No, no, no. We're going to treat the ulcer with antacids, because acid drills holes (and if you already have a hole, we'll patch it up!), and we're going to treat the heart disease with new arteries to bypass the rusty ones, because rust is no good.* But there was a voice out there somewhere, saying, "We don't understand this well enough yet."

Fortunately, some brave, brilliant folks were looking at infectious disease. God knows why. Maybe they were infectious disease specialists. Maybe they tripped over some old information. Maybe they were just hopelessly curious, as so many great scientists are. For whatever reason, a few individuals began to notice and report that people who had heart attacks had more positive culture results for *Chlamydia pneumoniae* than those who didn't. *C. pneumoniae* is a bacterium. You may remember from biology class that bacteria are single-cell organisms. Not all bacteria are bad. We depend on some of the bacteria in our bodies to do things for us. For example, there are bacteria in our colon that help us digest food. But some bacteria are indeed harmful, and they are called *pathogens*. They generate pathology. *Chlamydia pneumoniae* is a pathogen. It's a bacterium you really don't want in your body. Far more common than it's sexually transmitted cousin, chlamydia pneumonia is a staggeringly ubiquitous upper respiratory infection. It also likes to live in the walls of your coronary arteries. If *Chlamydia pneumoniae* causes heart attacks, then its presence in your body might help explain why someone with no family history and no obvious classical risk factors could suddenly have a heart attack. Once you start thinking along infectious disease lines, some puzzling aspects of the heart attack epidemic make sense.

For example, the heart attack rate is decreasing slowly. No one knows why exactly. The traditional explanation is that people are behaving better, eating better, exercising more. Well, doctors are cynics, and we know people don't usually behave better. People behave badly. They always have, and they always will. So what else could be causing the decline (this is a relative term, of course, because people are still dying of coronary heart disease by the millions).

A fascinating alternative explanation may be that the heart attack rate is following the typical course of a prolonged infectious epidemic. As more than one study has noted, the decline of deaths due to heart attack corresponds with the introduction and common use of antibiotics. That's one reason some doctors began looking at the relationship between bacteria and heart disease.

Chlamydia pneumoniae was first isolated in 1986 and found to be associated with a number of respiratory illnesses, including pneumonia. The first suggestion of a connection between *Chlamydia pneumoniae* and coronary artery disease occurred in Helsinki, Finland, in 1988, when one study revealed that men experiencing heart attack or severe coronary disease were 2.6 times more likely to be positive for *Chlamydia pneumoniae* than those who were negative. Since then, nearly two dozen major studies have found epidemiological evidence of a connection between *Chlamydia pneumoniae* and coronary heart disease. But what does *C. pneumoniae* do to the coronary arteries that causes so much trouble?

This brings us to the missing piece of the puzzle, the biological missing link: inflammation. Inflammation is the body's defense mechanism. It keeps us healthy. It's the weapon the immune system uses to overwhelm and destroy invaders such as nasty bacteria.

Inflammation isn't just one process. It's a complicated cascade of biological processes known as the *inflammatory response*. This is a mechanism, composed both of chemicals circulating in the blood and of specialized blood cells that enter the bloodstream and head toward areas where there are infecting organisms. This is the response of an entire army of defensive mechanisms in your body, drafted to confront an army of invaders and slaughter them. The slaughter can take different forms: invading cells are sometimes dissolved by powerful enzymes; or they're engulfed by the defending cells—some invaders are, literally, eaten to death.

The method of demise isn't really important. What matters is this: Where there is infection, there is inflammation.

Everybody knows what happens when the immune system falters (that's what happens to people with acquired immunodeficiency syndrome [AIDS]). Your immune system doesn't work; invaders get into your body and storm your defenses and kill you. So a healthy immune system and its weapon, inflammation, are essential to life.

But the inflammation weapon can also go terribly wrong in the other direction. On occasion it can begin to overreact, to rage out of control and destroy not just invading organisms but healthy tissue as well. Some bacteria seem particularly adept at making the immune system, and the inflammatory response, misfire. That's how they survive. They fight slow wars of attrition, never really winning and never really losing either. All the while immune cells and chemicals are crashing about, causing "collateral damage."

Chlamydia pneumonia seems to be an infection of this sort. We don't know just yet what it is about chlamydia that allows it to hang on in the walls of coronary arteries despite constant assault by the body's immune system. But it does. So where there is *Chlamydia pneumoniae* there is constant inflammation in the arterial wall. *C. pneumoniae* doesn't really make you feel very sick, but it infects arterial walls in sufficient force to make the immune system misfire and produce more inflammation than infection. To understand why this is a bad thing, and how it's related to coronary heart disease, you have to understand a little more about inflammation.

Inflammation marshals defending cells into an area of infection, and they produce what's often called the triad of inflammation: *calor, rubor*, and *dolor*—heat, redness, and pain. That's the signature of the body's immune system. We've all seen it. You have a boo-boo on your skin. That triggers an inflammatory response. It gets warm, it gets red, and it hurts. This stuff occurs *inside* your body as well, even though you don't see it or feel it. The inflammatory cells—the defenders of the body, the army of the night—are marching toward the infecting bacteria and trying to destroy them.

Bacteria, for their part, have evolved mechanisms for dealing with this assault; otherwise they wouldn't be around anymore. *Chlamydia pneumoniae*, for whatever reason, seem to be able to exist in an uneasy equilibrium with these invading cells. Some *Chlamydia pneumoniae* remain in the body even after being assaulted. Others are destroyed. And new chlamydia organisms are born from the ones that aren't destroyed. The process begins again. The immune system's war against chlamydia resembles a siege more than a blitzkrieg campaign. That means that there are always immune cells in the area doing what it is they do. The immune response in the arterial walls never stops.

Most of the time inflammation is an appropriate response, and it can prevent you from dying. Over millions of years of evolution, the inflammatory response has acquired certain characteristics that are lethal to bacteria. There are enzymes that are secreted by the inflammatory responding cells that are designed to harm tissue. These enzymes are supposed to dissolve bacteria. And that's often precisely what they do. Think about a boil that becomes infected and filled with pus. You know what that is? Dead bacteria soup! It's dead invading cells, enzymes, and pieces of bacteria, all minced together in a big dissolving muck. It's the inflammatory response at endgame, and although it may look and smell disgusting, that is precisely what should happen.

But this complex and delicately balanced process can go wrong. Ideally, when the bacteria are gone, and the stimulus for the inflammatory response has disappeared, you want the muck to go away. You want the soldiers to return to their barracks. If they hang around after the threat is gone, if they go into "siege mode," that's not a good thing, because then the soldiers get restless, and they do what they're programmed to do: They attack something. Sometimes that "something" is your own tissue. *"Hey, it's kind of a boring day today; let's secrete some enzymes! There's no bacteria here, so we'll go after some healthy tissue. You know what looks like a good target? This arterial wall right over here!"*

Theoretically the inflammatory cells should be able to operate safely in the walls of coronary arteries. The mechanism is finely tuned and quite elegant. But there is always a fine line when you kill anything that is biological in the human body, because our biological mechanisms and those of bacteria aren't all that different. The immune system is always looking for the edge—*"How can we kill a lot of bacteria with the least amount of damage to normal human tissue?"* The inflammatory response—*"I can secrete a little Lysol here, a little Drano there, and dissolve the bacteria. Of course, I'll probably put a couple of holes in the coronary artery, but we can always repair that when the bacteria go away. At least the bacteria will be gone, and we'll have won the war"*—is a very dangerous game. It's like bombing your own cities after they've been overrun by the enemy and planning to fix them after the enemy retreats.

Disturb the balance of the response a little, and the inflammatory response can cause disease and destruction of its own that might be worse than the trouble caused by the invading bacteria.

To some degree, this is exactly what's going on in coronary arteries that have been infected by *Chlamydia pneumoniae*. There is a decreased bacterial burden, and yet the inflammatory response persists far more powerfully than it should. These excess defender cells hang out in the arterial walls smoking cigarettes, reading the racing form, flipping coins, and doing other bad things. Mostly they induce inflammation. They induce heat. They induce swelling. *They dissolve healthy arterial wall tissue!*

How do we know this is happening, and how can we stop it? For me, the answers to those questions began to come into focus as I wrestled with the apparent contradictions of the patients I saw in the ICU—people who didn't fit the standard model of heart disease. These were the folks who had heart attacks despite having normal serum cholesterol levels, people who had heart attacks despite the absence of hard plaque, people with "normal" cardiogram results. I couldn't help but think that heart attack and progressive angina were in fact two separate diseases, and thus the ways you attacked both of them had to be different. Yes, they were related. They both occurred in the arteries of the heart, they both affected the muscle of the heart, they both gave you pain, and they both could kill you. Although the therapy for one might overlap in a gray area to be part of the therapy for the other, our specific plan for treating angina, or hard-plaque disease, was not preventing the other disease, heart attacks. And that's what was making me crazy.

I was fortunate, because I had the luxury of being a journalist as well as a doctor. Most doctors restrict their research and reading to topics that fall into their own particular area of expertise; I was expected to cast the net a bit wider. So it was that a few years back, I found myself at a string of conferences in which heart disease was the focus of attention. At a cardiology conference, that wouldn't be such a big surprise. But at a conference for infectious disease specialists? For diabetologists? For kidney specialists? At each of these conferences, I was informed by the novel approach of doctors whose lives were not necessarily spent treating heart attack patients. This was especially true on the day I walked into the American Diabetes Association meetings and heard Dr. Steven Nissen, a cardiologist at the Cleveland Clinic, talking to an audience of diabetes experts, talking not about blood sugar, but about heart disease, and a tiny ultrasound probe that he and his fellow researchers had inserted into the coronary arteries of their patients. What they saw was not the standard hard plaque that everyone knew was there, but something called "soft plaque." I perked up my ears. Soft plaque? A new and different kind of plaque? Not the stuff I had seen all those years ago in the autopsy suite? Not the stuff we were seeing on angiograms and not the stuff we were bypassing and angioplasting? What was this stuff? Nissen began to talk.

Dr. Nissen was present at a diabetes meeting because people with diabetes often die of heart disease. He was there to discuss the link between cholesterol and heart disease, but he studied this link in a novel way: He was using his ultrasound probe to see whether there was cholesterol in the artery wall that wasn't protruding into the center of the artery. Ultrasound is like a submarine's sonar gear. It bounces sound waves off the tissue layers that make up the thickness of the artery's walls and "listens" for their echoes. If there is extra fat in the wall, the echo is different from the echo if there isn't any. The machine then turns the echoes into pictures. His machine was giving him pictures of stuff that would be invisible on standard angiograms because his fatty deposits didn't make the artery "lumpy"; they just made its walls thicker.

He asked a simple question: *Is there more fat in these walls than we had previously thought, on the basis of the techniques we had used before?* And the answer he got was a resounding, *You bet!*

Nissen reported finding artery after artery loaded with fat. He displayed dramatic pictures taken in his catheter lab, pictures that showed pockets of stuff, presumably cholesterol, inside the arterial wall itself—not poking into the area where the blood flows, but just making the wall *fatter*. His point was that this didn't create a narrower opening, as typically happened with the accumulation of hard plaque, until the very end of the process. That solved part of the mystery. People with this kind of plaque wouldn't get angina. The blood was flowing just fine through their coronary arteries.

There are layers in an arterial wall, and what Nissen found was that as cholesterol accumulated between the layers, it didn't bulge into the opening and occlude the artery—as we would have seen on a standard angiogram—it bulged *out*. Think of it this way: If an artery is a doughnut, then hard plaque makes the doughnut hole smaller; soft plaque just makes the doughnut *thicker*. So you end up with a great big doughnut with a pretty normal sized hole.

This was the first lightbulb that went on for me, explaining, as it did, why people with normal angiograms, with normal "doughnut holes," and sometimes even with normal lipid profiles, still had trouble. They had plaque we couldn't see!

People with too much cholesterol in their blood were parking it in globs in their coronary artery walls. These were the globs we couldn't see with an angiogram. And they were present in people who thought their cholesterol levels were just fine. Wrong!

This plaque was interesting for another reason. It wasn't made of rock-hard calcium that would never go away. It was made mostly of jellylike stuff that might get absorbed back into the blood if you lowered the blood cholesterol level. More cholesterol in the blood, the plaque would get fatter; less cholesterol, the plaque would get smaller. That would explain why the diet gurus were having some success reducing people's heart attack risks.

That was the second lightbulb for me: Soft plaque was in equilibrium with the cholesterol in the blood; that would explain for the first time why lowering a person's cholesterol level would reduce his heart attack risk, even though it didn't change the size of the hard plaque already in his coronary arteries.

The United States is a nation that is drowning in cholesterol, and so we need to reexamine what it is we mean by the term *normal cholesterol*. Normal compared to what? Compared to everyone else who is dropping dead too early?

Nissen was one of the first to demonstrate why you could have a potentially lethal accumulation of plaque in your coronary arteries while exhibiting none of the classic symptoms of angina. He also pointed out that soft plaque was widespread in individuals of all ages, all sizes, all backgrounds. The point was not that everybody he studied had experienced a heart attack, but that he understood where cholesterol fit in the picture. He found in many of these people this so-called soft plaque, which he described as pathological—*not normal*—and which can lead to disease in the coronary arteries. That's one characteristic heart attack and angina have in common: It's a coronary artery issue. That this stuff was made of cholesterol seemed to imply that cholesterol was playing a very important role in soft plaque.

Nissen found soft plaque in 60 percent of the subjects between the ages of thirty and thirty-nine. Sixty percent! Even more shocking is the realization that standard angiography results were negative in 90 percent of the study's population. They showed no plaque. The patients should have been healthy. Subsequent research has confirmed Nissen's findings that coronary atheroma (plaque) is not only possible but likely, even when there is no visible blockage. And yet the hunt for soft plaque remains an afterthought in cardiac care. It's at least partly a technical problem. Even in patients who undergo cardiac catheterizations, intracoronary ultrasound is rarely, if ever, performed. It is a delicate and difficult study. It is still basically a research tool, not a screening test.

Then I attended a similar series of meetings for infectious disease specialists, where I was surprised to hear everyone talking about chronic inflammation, chronic infection, and how these two were connected to the risk of heart attack. Their focus was on *Chlamydia pneumoniae*, but there were other bacteria mentioned, too. The point was this: New research demonstrated that cultures taken from heart patients were growing bacteria! Did this make sense? Yes, because fat is an excellent food for bacteria. So now we had two pieces of the puzzle: cholesterol and something that really likes cholesterol, bacteria, living and growing together in an area where you don't want them, the coronary artery.

There were other meetings as well, and one after another they revealed tiny pieces of the puzzle. Together, they combined to form nothing less spectacular than a new model of heart disease. For me it was a head-slapping moment, the kind that makes you say *"How could we have been so blind?"* The truth is, we weren't blind. It takes an awful lot of hard, careful work, a lot of digging away, before everything makes sense. Many of the most brilliant discoveries in science have been like that. The incomprehensible becomes obvious only after a bunch of very bright people put all the evidence together in a way that makes it obvious. That's what happened here. Suddenly, with all this information on our plate, the explanation for heart attack becomes crystal clear: In a word, here it is:

Inflammation.

How do we know it's inflammation? Because we have the evidence. And if the evidence is correct, we have a new model for heart attack. It looks like this:

STEP 1 There's cholesterol in the blood, and some of this cholesterol, for reasons we don't understand completely, finds its way to the coronary arteries, where it forms soft plaque. Soft plaque is invisible to the normal arterial studies like the angiogram, and it doesn't cause symptoms. Over the course of time this soft plaque gets bigger and bigger.

STEP 2 *Lunch is served!* Into this soft plaque migrate bacteria; there they start growing and having a high old time. The most likely bacterial candidate here is *Chlamydia pneumoniae.*

STEP 3 The inflammatory response: Once the bacteria are sensed by the body, alarm bells go off in the form of chemical triggers, and into the walls of the coronary arteries gravitate cells that the body uses to get rid of bacteria: inflammatory cells. These cells start secreting chemicals and doing other things to destroy the invaders, and in the process there is always collateral damage. (By the way, it is interesting to note that there is literature to suggest that you don't necessarily need the bacteria to cause trouble: For reasons we don't completely understand, fat in the coronary artery, itself, can trigger the inflammatory response. Granted, there is almost certainly a hierarchy of badness: Cholesterol alone is bad, but in combination with *Chlamydia pneumoniae* or some other bacteria, it's even worse.)

The inflammatory response smolders on for weeks and months and years. In a way, it's an entirely appropriate response, yet in another way it's inappropriate. It's appropriate because the bacteria need to be destroyed. However, the collateral damage caused by the inflammatory cells, although perhaps acceptable in some parts of the body, is unacceptable in the coronary arteries. It doesn't matter whether you get a boil on your leg because eventually the boil pusses out—it opens and it drains and all that bad stuff floats away and you heal up and feel fine; that's the normal course of curing a skin infection. But think about that same process in your coronary arteries:

> Here come the inflammatory response cells. They're chewing away at the bacteria and the fat in the coronary artery. They're forming a "boil" in the wall of the artery. And where does the pus drain? Into the hole of the doughnut. It erodes through the wall! Suddenly the blood that is flowing seamlessly through this coronary artery is exposed to all the debris, the liquified fat, the dead and destroyed defending cells, the dead and destroyed bacteria, and this "soup" that is exposed to the blood supply is intensely thrombogenic, meaning it makes the blood clot. Just like that, within a brief period—seconds to minutes to hours— the blood turns to Jell-O and *bang!* The coronary artery is obstructed, and the blood flow that had been feeding the heart is now cut off behind a dam, behind a massive blood clot. Beyond that point the heart gets no blood. It literally suffocates and dies.

That is a heart attack, major or minor, depending on where the perforation occurs and how quickly the victim receives help, but a heart attack nonetheless.

This is our new model, and it makes perfect sense. It explains a lot, most notably why heart disease isn't always a gradual process—why you don't get a little sicker and a little sicker and then have a heart attack. Soft plaque doesn't protrude into the coronary artery, so blood flow can be relatively normal right up to the point when the soft plaque ruptures through the artery wall and all hell breaks loose. Then everything happens very quickly, and we all say, *"My God, where did that come from?"*

It's a chronic disease, of course; it's been going on for years. But it's a different kind of chronic disease, with a different set of symptoms, a different kind of presentation than what you would get from the kind of heart disease that causes angina. Angina is caused by hard plaque aggressively and visibly growing into the artery, causing limitations to blood flow and subsequent pain. The other type of heart disease is silently brewing in the arterial wall, waiting for a single moment when it can and will cause the greatest possible mischief. And when that moment occurs, it's catastrophic.

So, what do we do? How do we fight this invisible enemy? It's hardly practical to suggest intracoronary ultrasounds for everyone—they're far too invasive and dangerous and expensive. But there is a marker for inflammation. It's called *C-reactive protein*, and it has been shown to be a powerful indicator for people at a high risk for heart disease. C-reactive protein can be measured through a simple test, and it's my feeling that, given current research, there is no reason not to be tested for C-reactive protein. Just as you should know your cholesterol numbers, you should know whether your body's inflammatory response is in high gear (we'll discuss the C-reactive protein issue in greater detail later, in the testing chapter). Of course, the two are linked. If you reduce the level of cholesterol in your blood, you'll reduce the inflammation and, hence, the level of C-reactive protein. The point is to understand the model and attack the disease on as many fronts as possible. We want to lower cholesterol level not only through diet and exercise, but through the use of statins. We want to reduce inflammation through the use of aspirin. And, finally, we want to make sure the body is free of infectious disease. If bacteria are present, antibiotics should be used.

Why each of these components is necessary and effective will be examined in subsequent chapters. For now, the most important point to understand is this: We have a new model. It's logical and provides the basis for a course of treatment. In the past, without this explanation we couldn't get to the root cause of the problem. We were guessing. We treated the angina and you felt better. We had you exercise and you felt better. We took away your cigarettes, encouraged you to lose weight, and so forth. We made everybody *feel* better on the way to the grave- yard, but we didn't attack the real problem. Now, for the first time, not only can we make you feel better, and wiggle your death rate a little, but we can make an astounding statement:

We can slow the clock on death.

CHAPTER FOUR

Aspirin

We're going to talk about aspirin first because it's simply the most amazing drug you can imagine. It's also one of the oldest. To give you some idea of just how impressive a drug it is, consider this: When I was a medical student, a popular teaching tool involved a hypothetical scenario in which we, the students, were asked to pick five drugs we would want to have at our disposal if we ever found ourselves stranded on a desert island. And, of course, we would have to defend each choice.

Four of these drugs, in no particular order, usually turned out to be penicillin, morphine, insulin, and some type of diuretic. But the unanimous winner, the number one choice, without question, was aspirin. It's that powerful, that reliable, that versatile. Aspirin is an analgesic, meaning it relieves pain. It's an anti-inflammatory drug (technically it falls into a class of drugs called the nonsteroidal anti-inflammatories), which means it has the ability to reduce redness, swelling, and heat. And it has anticoagulant properties. Back then, we really didn't even know much about its ability to help prevent heart attacks; we just knew the darn thing worked and it worked in all sorts of areas. Aspirin was like the Swiss army knife of drugs. (It's interesting to note, too, that of all the drugs we agreed to take with us to this fictitious desert island, not one was invented after 1950. Despite all of our vast medical knowledge, with all the wonderful new drugs at our disposal—and many are indeed spectacular—it's hard to get the same bang for your buck that you get with some of the old standbys.) So dust off your aspirin bottle, because it can do wonders.

Aspirin is derived from a chemical found in willow bark and other natural sources. People have known about the amazing benefits of chewing willow bark for thousands of years. Hippocrates used willow leaves to control pain (he advised women in labor to chew them).

The secret of willow may have been lost to formal western medicine for a millennium or so, but there is evidence that it was used continuously as a popular folk remedy throughout Europe from the time of Hippocrates until the eighteenth century.

It was "rediscovered" in 1763 when the Reverend Edward Stone of Chipping Norton in Oxfordshire, England, wrote a letter to the Royal Society:

> "Among the many useful discoveries which this age has made, there are very few which better deserve the attention of the public than what I am about to lay before your lordship. There is a bark of an English tree, which I have found by experience to be a powerful astringent, and very efficacious in curing aguish and intermittent disorders."

The reverend's letter created a sensation. The question of the day became "What is it about willow that cures fever, reduces aches and pains, and stops the shivers (ague) of disease?"

Although Reverend Stone was English, it was the Germans who solved the riddle of willow. Some of the best chemists of the day worked at the Pharmacologic Institute of Munich. It was there, in 1828, that the active ingredient of willow, salicin, was first isolated. The stuff looked funny; it was yellow. And it tasted terrible. It was so bitter, in fact, that many people vomited trying to swallow it.

By 1830 the French had reduced three pounds of willow bark to one ounce of salicin. That was an awful lot of bark for very little active ingredient. Other groups looked for better sources in other plants. Wintergreen turned out to be rich in salicylic acid. But everyone in Europe, it seemed, was looking for a way to make cheap salicylic acid in a test tube.

Although the French, Germans, and English competed feverishly (yes, the pun was intended), it was the Germans who won again. They produced a pure cheap synthetic product in 1860.

But the stuff still tasted terrible, upset people's stomachs, and induced vomiting. Then, in 1898—still not even the twentieth century!—came the most famous and important development of all. Felix Hoffmann (you guessed it, another German chemist), working for the Bayer Corporation, had been searching for a form of salicylic acid that was clinically effective but also well tolerated by the human body. In that year he invented a chemically altered version he called . . . aspirin. Why aspirin? "A" from A (cetyl), a chemical, and "Spir" from Spir (aea), a natural plant source of salicylic acid. After that, predictably, all hell broke loose. Scores of competitors entered the field, the market exploded, and aspirin became the wonder drug that it remains today.

That's the basic, abbreviated history of aspirin. We know people have been using plant derivatives to treat illnesses for ages, so it's highly unlikely that the use of salicylates began only when people started writing about them. The fact that Hippocrates knew about it suggests that aspirin (in one form or another) is one of the oldest drugs known to humankind.

As old and seemingly simple as it is, however, aspirin is in fact a remarkably wondrous and complex drug. Even today, after hundreds of years of careful scientific research and chemical evolution, we still don't know everything that aspirin does; we're not sure of all its many properties. What we are sure of is that a number of those properties are extraordinarily powerful and beneficial. The more you study aspirin, the more amazing it seems: You find, almost by coincidence, that you prescribe it for one condition, and, lo and behold, it does something else good while it's doing what you originally wanted it to do.

To that end, doctors began prescribing aspirin to combat heart disease some years ago. The first time I had an inkling that aspirin was part of the anti–heart attack mix was shortly after I finished medical school, when I received some cryptic information from a cardiologist. I said to him, in passing: "Suppose someone is having a heart attack at home. How would you advise this person to get to the hospital?" I expected the cardiologist to say: "Get an ambulance, you idiot! Don't let the patient drive himself!" But that wasn't what I meant, and it wasn't the first thing the cardiologist said. The very first words out of his mouth were "Tell him to take an aspirin."

"Huh?" I said. "Aspirin?"

The cardiologist nodded. "That's right. Before you do anything else, tell him to take an aspirin."

Having never heard anything like this before, and having never read anything about it in the popular literature, I was confused. But the more I listened, the more I began to hear the same advice. It became something of a mantra among cardiologists in the late 1970s, despite the fact that it hadn't yet seeped into the popular medical literature. Cardiologists who saw a lot of patients with heart attacks were becoming convinced that aspirin had some beneficial result. And they were right.

Not that they thoroughly understood the mechanism for this benefit. Their best guess was very straightforward and stemmed from the commonly accepted belief that heart attacks are caused by blood clots. The reason for the blood clot is irrelevant. They knew only that many patients suffered heart attacks because of blood clots in the coronary arteries, so their logical, mechanistic thinking was, *Let's give these patients a drug that can prevent the blood from clotting.* Well, aspirin's anticoagulant properties had been identified nearly a century earlier, so it seemed to be a sensible candidate for the job.

Aspirin prevents blood from clotting by turning off one of the components in the blood that help form clots, the platelets. Blood clots form through two different mechanisms. One is humeral—that is, there are chemicals in the blood that form little jellylike complexes, effectively turning the blood into Jell-O. The other mechanism is the platelet mechanism. Platelets are called *platelets* because, believe it or not, they look like tiny plates under the microscope. They are "tiny protoplasmic disks, smaller than red blood cells, that are found in the blood and help promote coagulation" (*Webster's*). Obviously, it makes sense for you to have these things in your bloodstream. If there is a hole in your blood vessel, you would like to plug that hole before you bleed to death. Platelets are attracted to areas of vascular injury. Presumably this property was extremely useful back in our caveman days, when such holes were common—gaping wounds caused by rocks, spears, saber-toothed tiger bites, and the like. When the platelets sense there is a vascular injury, they attach themselves to the injury site and then attach themselves to each other, creating a platelet plug. The body quite literally puts a cork on itself. This is the first stage of the clotting process: platelets holding the fort while the humeral mechanism forms the Jell-O-like clot that eventually (ideally) stops the flow of blood permanently. Like fixing a leaky bicycle tire, it's a plug-and-patch process.

Unfortunately, the clotting mechanism isn't always a good thing. It can go awry and plug up areas that really shouldn't be plugged up. When platelets plug up the coronary arteries, choking off the flow of blood to the heart, it's a very bad thing indeed. So thirty years ago, wizened cardiologists were saying that if you gave aspirin to a heart attack patient and prevented the platelets from forming plugs, the coronary arteries wouldn't be obstructed. It seemed to make sense.

This led, predictably, to the question of whether this effect would result in a risk of bleeding elsewhere. The honest answer was, Yes. But the risk/benefit ratio here was death versus the small risk of bleeding elsewhere, so both patient and doctor said, in essence, *"We'll take it!"*

Used this way, aspirin was immediately found to be remarkable for a number of reasons. First of all, only a very small dose was required for it to be effective. Second, its anti-platelet activity was irreversible. That's why it was commonly given to patients who had been stricken at home. You took one tablet, you let it get absorbed into the blood at home while you were getting ready to go to the hospital, and almost instantaneously the platelet activity was turned off—permanently. The body would have to create another whole population of platelets in order to be able to form effective platelet plugs again. If you find it difficult to picture this scenario—if you think of a heart attack as being a catastrophic, violent event that renders its victim limp and usually lifeless—you're not alone. But the truth is, most heart attacks aren't "sudden-death" events (although, obviously, they can be). Most involve less severe symptoms, such as sudden, severe chest pain or an overall sense of feeling "funny." There can be tingling in the extremities, lightheadedness, and an assortment of other unpleasant symptoms. Usually, there is time to react, and to think about a course of action.

The first step, cardiologists agreed, was to turn off the platelet activity. The fact that this worked—that it did, in fact, seem temporarily to prevent heart attacks from killing you— naturally led doctors to wonder whether aspirin might be effective in the overall war against heart disease.

Their thinking was rational: They were giving aspirin to patients who were having acute heart attacks, and when they did so, they found that it was an astoundingly good drug, that it did ameliorate symptoms and save lives. The numbers were (and are) incredible. Aspirin was unquestionably, irrefutably a miracle drug in that sense. It not only gave you time to get to the hospital, but once you were there, we discovered, all the drugs we could give you, all the interventions at our disposal, were still helped by that first dose of aspirin. If that was the only thing that aspirin did to your heart, it would still have been the MVP of heart drugs. It was cheap, it was easy to make, it was relatively nontoxic, and it provided a tremendous benefit: It literally saved your life. Not a bad drug.

So cardiologists began to prescribe aspirin for that reason alone. After all, it was a short step in the rationale to move from "Aspirin can make a heart attack less severe by making the blood-clotting mechanism less troublesome" to the next level, which was "Maybe if we turned off the platelets to begin with, then the heart attack wouldn't occur in the first place." This, too, was a reasonable assumption, and indeed aspirin did seem to be effective when prescribed in a preventative manner. The first group of patients to benefit, naturally, were those deemed to be at the greatest risk, because they had the most to lose. You don't give a drug with potential side effects to someone for whom it's not going to do any good, but rather to someone whose heart is a ticking time bomb, someone who is waiting for a second heart attack. If you have a drug that has some acknowledged risk, but a potential benefit of saving the patient's life, then you give the drug and see what happens. For that reason, the next wave in the cardiac literature involved large population-based studies asking the question "If you take an aspirin a day, every day, after your first heart attack, can it prevent you from having a second heart attack?" Here, again, the research was very clear. It can. There were dramatic reductions in the rate at which these patients suffered second heart attacks.

The results, although encouraging, were also somewhat perplexing, for we still didn't really understand why aspirin worked on these patients. It was prescribed because doctors thought aspirin could prevent the formation of platelet plugs and blood clots, but the more fundamental question "Why is the blood clotting?" remained unanswered. After all, platelets need a trigger to start their activity; they don't spontaneously clot.

The first suggested answer was "Vessel injury caused these platelets to clot." What injury? Well, maybe those calcified plaques appear to be a vessel injury to a few confused platelets. The platelets clumped, they formed a plug, and the clotting cascade began.

But that model didn't explain what first triggered the mechanism. In other words, one day you've got a great, hulking piece of calcium in your coronary artery, and the platelets and red blood cells and white blood cells are slipping by without any trouble. The next day the platelets think this calcium is a saber-toothed tiger bite and they decide in their very binary way to take some action.

We do lots of things in medicine without understanding how they work. It's enough (though intellectually unsatisfying) to know they do something good. But lack of understanding should produce some caution. Give aspirin, but with a healthy dose of "I don't know why."

As it turned out, the "I don't know" was important, for it led to speculation about what might happen if aspirin were prescribed in an attempt to prevent not just second heart attacks but first heart attacks. In other words, "Why wait for a heart attack before you approve the use of aspirin? After all, that first heart attack can kill you." That's a much more difficult question to answer ethically. To be truthful, that's what this was: a question of ethics. Because although it's very easy to design a study with a drug that has some side effects if you're going to use that drug to save the lives of people at risk of death—that is, people who have already suffered one heart attack—what do you do with people who have never had a heart attack, people for whom the risk/benefit ratio is more controversial? If everyone walking down the street took an aspirin, a certain percentage would have an allergic reaction, another group would bleed from an ulcer, another would have a tendency to bruise more easily—all because their platelets had been turned off. And not all of these folks would have ever had a heart attack, even if they never took an aspirin in their life.

That's one reason that it took a long time for these studies to be undertaken—in fact, many are still in the process of being completed—but there is ample evidence to support the notion that aspirin is highly effective in the prevention of first heart attacks, as well as second heart attacks. Again, however, the question *Why?* arises. Why does aspirin work? Why are these platelets cruising along one moment, minding their own business, and then suddenly clumping up and causing a heart attack the next moment?

Under the old model of heart disease, you couldn't find a trigger. Although aspirin was useful, and it solved some of the puzzle, it didn't explain all of it. Aspirin's benefits were out of proportion to its platelet effects. What else was in the mix? What was it about aspirin that made it more effective than other antiplatelet drugs, such as ibuprofen and a whole host of other nonsteroidal anti-inflammatory drugs, or even other far more powerful blood thinners, such as Coumadin? If the platelet model of aspirin's effect was the only mechanism of action, then these other drugs should have been at least as effective as aspirin, if not better, for they were much stronger. But that's not the way it worked. For example, when we examined the effect of Coumadin, which was the easiest and safest of the anticoagulant drugs for an outpatient to use, and compared it to the effect of aspirin in terms of preventing heart attack, aspirin was the winner, hands down!

Naturally, this led to the assumption that aspirin must be doing something other than just turning off platelets, that it has additional properties that somehow contribute to the prevention of heart attacks. What could they be? Well, remember that for the longest time aspirin had been considered effective in relieving ague, the shivers and chills associated with high fever and inflammation. The common cold produces ague, as does the flu. Additionally, we've known since the middle of the nineteenth century that aspirin is one of the most potent drugs in fighting rheumatic fever, as it remains to this day. Rheumatic fever is a disease characterized by inflammation. Throughout the twentieth century, in fact, there were observations that aspirin is particularly effective at cooling down the inflammation caused by a variety of autoimmune disorders. Was it, then, perhaps the anti-inflammatory aspect of aspirin, described so often and so vividly centuries before, that was actually causing this mysterious improvement in the primary heart attack rate? Was it aspirin's ability to relieve ague, rather than it's anticoagulation effect, that made it such a wonderful, heart-saving drug?

Think about it. Why should you have to turn off platelets unless something odd is turning them on? That sudden mysterious platelet-inciting factor was the part that always stuck in my craw. Then we began to find evidence for inflammation in the coronary arteries leading to disease, and it all started to make sense. Inflammation turns on platelets. Aspirin turns off inflammation.

The evidence that aspirin works by cooling off the inflammatory response began to mount up. For example, aspirin prevents heart attacks in people who don't have obvious preexisting heart disease. Again, this fits the model of inflammation leading to heart attack. Now, I must add a caveat here. The empirical evidence for primary protection is very new, but the data we have so far are quite powerful and quite convincing.

To paraphrase Groucho: "I'm going to ask my cardiologist if he's taking an aspirin a day. If he says no, I'm going to find another cardiologist."

There are other characteristics of aspirin that mesh nicely with the anti-inflammatory model, one of the most interesting of which is our old friend C-reactive protein. C-reactive protein, you'll recall, is a marker for inflammation, and what aspirin does in people with elevated levels of C-reactive protein is make the C-reactive protein level go down, reliably. So here again we have the inflammatory model, which explains why people without obvious heart disease as measured by angiogram get heart attacks. We have an inflammatory model that explains why C-reactive protein level goes up in people at risk, and we have a model that explains why an anti-inflammatory drug, aspirin, makes conditions better.

Aspirin turns down the inflammatory response, which is the eventual reason platelets are activated and form blood clots. Aspirin has a one-two knockout punch: It turns off the platelets, and it turns off what drives the platelets to clot! So I ask you again, Is that not a wonder drug?

Here's part of an editorial that appeared in the *American Journal of Cardiology* on July 1, 2002 (vol. 90, no. 1), one that strongly supports the notion that the increased use of aspirin is contributing to a decrease in the rate of heart attack:

> Increasing emphasis on the role of inflammation in the development of atherosclerosis and plaque stability raises the intriguing possibility that the benefits of aspirin are partially mediated by modification of inflammatory processes—an example of the wheel turning full circle. Supportive evidence is provided by studies of aspirin for the primary and secondary prevention of ischemic heart disease. Plasma C-reactive protein (CRP) level is a good indicator of coronary risk, and when high, as in patients with symptomatic coronary artery disease, the effect of aspirin in reducing CRP levels, even in the low doses currently used in cardiovascular medicine, is quite impressive. . . .
>
> In the interim, it is back to good old aspirin—tried, trusted, and faithful—even if 100 years after its initial use we still are unsure as to why it is so effective. Nonetheless . . . we must conclude there is no better single oral platelet inhibitor available than aspirin for the long-term

management of patients with acute and chronic coronary disease.

If you'd like numbers to support this thesis, here are just a few. A five-year follow-up of the Physician's Health Study, involving 22,071 male physicians in the United States, turned up these results: Compared to physicians who took placebo in a double-blind study, those physicians who took 325 milligrams of aspirin per day (one adult tablet) experienced a 44 percent decrease in the risk of heart attack! That's not just an impressive result; that's a nuclear-weapon-grade result. If this study is accurate, and I have no reason to believe it is not, then you give yourself a 44 percent edge in the war against heart disease simply by popping an aspirin a day.

There are studies to suggest that some of the other nonsteroidal anti-inflammatories have some effect on the risk of heart attack, but aspirin at this point seems to be uniquely effective. An editorial in the *American Heart Journal* in March 2002 (vol. 143, no. 3) asked: "Aspirin: Redundant in users of nonaspirin, nonsteroidal antiinflammatory agents?" The answer, research indicates, is no. Aspirin is such a unique drug that even if you are taking another drug, such as ibuprofen, you still need aspirin to reduce your heart attack risk.

Efficacy aside, there are other reasons to use aspirin. It's relatively safe, it's relatively cheap, and you don't need much of it. The question then becomes, How much is enough? There have been studies that have compared a broad spectrum of dosages, and the most reliable seem to indicate that you really don't need more than about 100 milligrams per day. That's a very small amount. Many doctors are recommending that a single baby aspirin may be enough to protect most people from the risk of heart attack.

Admittedly, aspirin (like any drug) is not for everyone. It has some potential side effects, almost all of which end if you simply stop taking it or reduce the dosage. The one that causes most problems and is the most common is bleeding—either gastrointestinal or cerebral. It's understandable that a drug that turns off platelets will make you more susceptible to bleeding in case of injury. In fact, the literature is replete with studies showing that people on aspirin have a slightly increased risk of bleeding ulcers and other gastrointestinal disorders, as well as a very small increase—but definitely an increase—in risk of hemorrhagic stroke.

The question then becomes, "Oh, my God, if I'm going to have a stroke, is it worth doing this to protect my heart?!" As with anything else in medicine, the answer once again lies with the risk/benefit ratio: how many people would have died of a heart attack if they weren't taking aspirin versus how many people had trouble with stroke while taking aspirin. The statistics overwhelmingly favor taking aspirin to drop the heart attack risk. That is to say, more people will die, more people will be injured, more people will be incapacitated because they did not take aspirin and thus had heart attacks than would be injured by stroke. So although the stroke potential shouldn't be ignored, neither should it serve as a blanket excuse not to take aspirin.

People who have any sort of bleeding disorder have what is called a *relative contraindication* to using blood thinners or drugs that provoke bleeding. For this reason, people with known ulcer disease used to be told they couldn't take aspirin; however, that was before we knew what really caused many ulcers, which is the bacterium *H. pylori*. But if you can cure the patient's *H. pylori*, then even a person who has a history of ulcer disease may be able to take aspirin. Conversely, there are some people taking aspirin who probably should be tested for *H. py-*

lori, at least if they have any intention of remaining on aspirin therapy for the rest of their lives. Certainly anyone who has a history of ulcer disease should be checked for *H. pylori* before embarking on a program of aspirin therapy—that's just common sense. All that being said, there is now plenty of evidence to show that in those people who no longer have a problem with *H. pylori*, aspirin is acceptable.

The appropriate question to ask here is, Of the people taking aspirin—otherwise healthy, without a history of gastrointestinal bleeding—how many of them actually bled? The answer is, Virtually no one. Aspirin is an extraordinarily safe drug, especially in the meager dosages we've been talking about. Unfortunately, aspirin has had a bad rap in recent years because of other nonsteroidal anti-inflammatories, all of which will predispose you to bleeding. (Acetaminophen [Tylenol], by the way, is not a nonsteroidal anti-inflammatory drug and offers no benefit in our model of heart disease even though it is a painkiller. Part of the reason doctors and patients are wary of aspirin has been a very successful marketing campaign for acetaminophen that points out that it is less likely to upset your stomach than aspirin is. That may be true, though there is some evidence to the contrary. But it also won't cure your heart disease. I could drink a bottle of tap water a day and it also wouldn't upset my stomach or cause me to bleed.)

Nonsteroidal anti-inflammatories can cause a host of other complications. Some people are allergic to aspirin. It can cause problems with asthma. It can cause or exacerbate kidney problems. All nonsteroidal anti-inflammatories, in fact, carry the risk of some kidney damage, especially in people who are dehydrated. An obvious group of people likely to be prone to dehydration are people who are being given diuretics for heart failure.

Then there's the question of drug interactions with aspirin, specifically with a group of antihypertensive drugs called the *angiotensin-converting enzyme* (ACE) *inhibitors*. Hundreds of thousands, if not millions, of Americans, take ACE inhibitors, primarily because of heart disease or heart failure. For these people, the most pressing concern is whether aspirin has a negative impact on the heart-sparing effect of ACE inhibitors—taking aspirin along with an ACE inhibitor may be throwing out the baby with the bath water, as it were. Does it make sense to prescribe aspirin to someone using an ACE inhibitor if indeed the aspirin limits the effectiveness of the ACE inhibitor, or worse, the combination of the two drugs is actually harmful?

A fair question; again, though, there is no simple answer. The most recent literature on this subject is mixed but seems to come down on the side of aspirin, for two reasons: (1) we are using aspirin to prevent death, a dramatic and clearly desirable result; and (2) we're talking about very small dosages of aspirin, as compared to some laboratory tests focusing on the aspirin–ACE inhibitor interaction. People who are on ACE inhibitors ought to check with the doctor before making a final decision. But in all likelihood, the recommendation will be to go ahead and take the aspirin.

There are considerations, too, for anyone already taking a prescription anticoagulant, such as Coumadin, as well as some oral diabetes drugs. Because aspirin may decrease the effect of drugs that rid the body of uric acid, taking it could affect gout therapy. Alcohol can be a problem with aspirin, too. And if you're using corticosteroids, such as prednisone or cortisone, aspirin could increase your risk of bleeding. The bottom line to all of this is rather simple and straightforward: If you're on a prescription drug, you should consult your physician before embracing a program of aspirin therapy.

Remember, there are a lot of contraindications in the world. If you open the *Physician's Desk Reference*, which is basically "The Doctor's Big Drug Book," and you throw a dart into a random page, then read the warnings associated with that drug, well, you'll probably just close the book and go home. You'd never prescribe or take any medication because every drug carries with it a list of warnings and caveats longer than the Hippocratic Oath. The lawyers wrote most of them. I'll bet a lot of lawyers are taking an aspirin a day.

You have to consider two different kinds of contraindications, absolute and relative. An *absolute contraindication* is one that says, NEVER EVER TAKE THIS DRUG THIS WAY. A *relative contraindication* is more like a PROCEED WITH CAUTION IF YOU'RE GOING TO TRY THIS DRUG sign. Some of these published risks should be weighed against the potential benefits the drugs offer. Most of the aspirin contraindications are *relative contraindications*.

In the pursuit of saving lives, I am willing to recommend that people take aspirin not only because the side effects are small in number, but because, in terms of their impact, those side effects are not often significant or debilitating. If you take an aspirin and you bleed—and at low dosages that is not likely to happen—well, we can fix that most of the time. If you lose a life, we can't give you another one.

I am not opposed to methodical and correct medical research. Neither am I opposed to being certain, beyond a reasonable doubt, that a particular course of treatment is effective. But I am opposed to sitting on my hands and waiting while the medical bureaucracy grinds out position papers and then slowly begins to disseminate the stuff they already know is true, even as an entire generation of Americans misses out on the benefits. And I'm tired of the FDA's requiring years of bureaucratic paper shuffling to recommend something trivial.

This book is being published on the cutting edge because it's not a journal for doctors to puzzle over. It's intended for you, the person who needs it *right now*! Aspirin fights inflammation and inflammation probably causes heart attacks. Arm yourself with this information. Talk with your doctor, if you'd like. And then make your own decision.

CHAPTER FIVE

Statins

Some pills are merely good for you, but statins are great for you. They will keep you alive.

The statins are a group of drugs that can lower your cholesterol level dramatically. They are relatively new, but you've already heard of them. Zocor (simvastatin) is one. So is Lipitor (atorvastatin). There are others. One is not even a prescription drug. As good as these drugs are, we have just scratched the surface of their potential benefits. We don't use them enough, and too few people are taking them right now.

If you want to live longer you will start taking a statin right now, even if your doctor tells you your heart disease risk is "low." What I'm offering is revolutionary advice. It is controversial. It is not the recommendation of the politically correct medical establishment. But it will be.

If you wait for the FDA and organized medicine to give you permission to save your own life, you may die waiting!

·····

Very early in my medical career, when I was just an intern, I took care of patients who suffered from high blood pressure. I routinely treated these people as if they were naughty children. I would put them on the most restrictive diets I could imagine: no salt, no fat, no this, no that—anything and everything to control their hypertension. When they returned for another round of tests, and their blood pressure readings were actually higher rather than lower, I responded with shock and amazement. I took it as a personal affront that these patients were not recovering.

"Are you eating salt?" I asked. "Are you following my instructions?" They shrugged their shoulders, scuffed the floor, averted their eyes, and eventually acknowledged their transgressions.

"I tried," they'd say. "But I really needed my french fries."

To this I would respond with a lengthy diatribe about living longer and being healthy. I would scold and chastise and generally act like the most brilliant, egotistical doctor in the world. The very thought of it now makes me cringe. Here I was, a twenty-six-year-old know-it-all, yelling and stomping my feet: "Does your life mean nothing to you? Don't you care about your children?!" I would muster all the moral authority that centuries of medical wisdom could give me, and all the textbook learning, and all the self-righteous indignation that only a twenty-six-year-old could have, and here were these people at sixty years of age, seventy years of age, coming in and telling me they couldn't stay away from a little french fry? I was appalled.

"You're old enough to know better," I'd say. And, of course, they were old enough to know better. They did know better. I was just too young to know it. They were making a decision, consciously or unconsciously, that the *quality* of their life was as important as the *quantity* of their life. They were saying to me, sometimes nonverbally, that they knew they should eat less salt, but avoiding it made their life difficult, and sometimes eating salt was a good thing (or at least an enjoyable thing), and eating cholesterol was a good thing, and they really didn't want to live the monastic life that I was trying to create for them. It might have been good for me, or even for most people, but not for them, not all the time.

One day I was approached by a senior staff member at the clinic where I worked. He was an attending physician, and part of his job was to peek over my shoulder once in a while, ask a few questions, and generally make sure I knew what I was doing.

"Salgo, I'm looking at your charts and watching you deal with these folks, and I notice you're not getting control of their blood pressure," he said.

My response to this accusation was a classic example of what medical people often do when events do not turn out exactly as they should: I blamed the patient.

"Well, I told them what to do, and they're not going to do it." I whined.

The attending physician shrugged. "Well, then you're not getting it done."

He was correct. Whatever the cause, if the patient is not re-sponding, then to some degree it's my fault as the doctor, not your fault as the patient, because a doctor should use any and all techniques at his disposal to get the desired effect to save people's lives. I hadn't yet learned that lesson; I hadn't learned that rigidity was a character flaw.

"But they won't stop eating this bad stuff!" I shouted.

With that, the attending physician smiled, looked me straight in the eye, and said, quite calmly, "Nor will they." This was something of a revelation to me. I mean, I was their doctor, for

God's sake. How could they *not* obey my orders? "These are human beings," the attending physician added. "And like all human beings, they prefer to enjoy their life."

"So what do you suggest? That we just let them die?"

He sighed, almost exasperated at my pigheadedness. "Just give them a blood pressure pill, okay?"

"But that's a pill."

"Uh-huh. What's so bad about that?"

I knew what I wanted to say: *My God, man, it's just not necessary! We can do this through diet and exercise. We can save these people naturally! If they'll only listen to me!* But what came out of my mouth was this: "I don't know."

The attending physician nodded. "Important career tip: You'll never know, because there is nothing bad about it. The entire development of twentieth-century medicine has led to the creation of this drug. When you take it, your blood pressure goes down. And once in a while you can still go to McDonald's."

"But McDonald's is bad!" I shouted.

Exasperated, he held up a finger of admonishment. Suddenly I was the naughty child.

"No, it isn't bad," he said. "It just isn't good. It contributes to high blood pressure in some people. But you know what? We can fix that for them. Sometimes, we can let them have their fries and have low blood pressure, too."

A lightbulb went on for me that day, and in its glow a good deal of my arrogance melted away. (Now that I think about it, lightbulbs are always going on for me. I must have come from a pretty dark place. Things are much brighter these days.) I stopped treating every patient in the same manner, stopped pretending that they could all be plugged into the same textbook formula. With some people I encouraged strict dietary guidelines; others I placed on antihypertension medication. Both groups saw their blood pressure decrease, and both found greater enjoyment in their lives. As for me, I became a different type of doctor, and, I hope, a better one.

I tell this story not merely as an act of penance, but as illustration of a point. I'm not advocating self-destructive, self-indulgent behavior. I'm simply acknowledging what you already know: that people are people and they will do what they do. I'm saying you don't have to live like a monk in order to save your own life. So many people out there in the self-help and "wellness" universe are preaching that unless you take draconian measures to change your lifestyle, you are going to get heart disease and die a terrible, stroke-infested death. I'm here to tell you that although they may be right, they also may be wrong. You see, there is a middle ground. You don't have to wear a robe and get a tonsure to live to the age of ninety. As with hypertension, there are drugs that help you control both the level and type of cholesterol in your body. And cholesterol, we now know, is the root of all evil when it comes to heart disease.

We all have choices that are within our power to make. You can choose to affect your cholesterol level with diet and diet alone, or you can choose to augment that diet with medication or with herbals (which are in fact medications that are not produced by drug companies but often have similar effects, as we'll discuss in a later chapter). You can choose to ignore my advice completely. It's up to you.

There's another thing you need to know before you make this decision, though, and that is this: Cholesterol is not entirely bad. Cholesterol is a fatty substance used by the body to make chemicals that are essential to life; there are, in fact, lots of chemicals in the body that must attach themselves to a fat in order to exist, and many of these use cholesterol as their foundation. You can make a lot of things out of cholesterol; it's sort of the Silly Putty of the body's chemicals. There are plenty of important life-giving chemicals that use cholesterol as a substrate, including bile, nerve tissue, and brain tissue. Cholesterol has acquired a bad reputation, but in reality it serves a vital purpose in human physiological processes. That said, it's also true that too much cholesterol, above and beyond what the body needs, is not a good thing, because excess cholesterol inevitably takes up residence in places where it can do harm.

When cholesterol accumulates in those places where it's stored without function, such as the coronary arteries, it causes mischief. Raw cholesterol combines with substances such as calcium to form plaque, and, as we've discussed, it can also form the mushy substance that sits within the artery walls, the soft plaque. Either way, it's nasty stuff. The cholesterol that is associated with soft plaque attracts other bad actors—bacteria, for instance, and cells that lead to the inflammatory response, cells called *foam cells*, and other inflammatory response cells, which eventually lead to the liquidization of the substances in this plaque. This liquid, this toxic soup, drills down through the coronary artery wall, causes a hole, and then spills into the coronary artery. This process leads to platelet aggregation, blood clot, and, in the worst-case scenario, heart attack and death. But it all starts, we think, with the accumulation and storage of what can only be termed *excess cholesterol.*

The assumption, if you listen only to the fad diet advertisements and to some of the "experts" talking about diets, is that all the cholesterol in your body enters through the food you eat, and that's just plain wrong. A lot of the cholesterol in the body—most of it, in fact—is from the body's own cholesterol-making factory, which turns out to be the liver. You can, to a degree, affect the total amount of cholesterol in your blood, which happens to be the cholesterol that seems to play the greatest role in the risk of heart disease, by changing your diet. If you eat a diet that is dramatically lower in cholesterol and fats, then you can make your total blood cholesterol level go down. In some people, cholesterol can be reduced to low-risk levels with diet alone. But for a great many people a diet change is just not enough. You can dramatically change your diet, eliminate almost all saturated fats, exercise like crazy, take all the "wiggle room" cholesterol out of your body, and your cholesterol level can still be too high.

That's because no matter what you do, the liver continues to crank out cholesterol. The liver is nothing less than a cholesterol machine, churning out roughly 80 percent of the body's cholesterol (the other 20 percent or so is probably diet-dependent). That 80 percent has nothing to do with diet or lifestyle. It is what it is. Genetically speaking, it's the hand you were dealt. In some people that 80 percent represents a modest amount of cholesterol, and those people aren't likely to have trouble modulating their total serum cholesterol level. Others aren't so fortunate. Regardless of what they eat, they're going to have trouble. If you fall into this category—if your cholesterol level is tremendously high—even if you take the 20 percent that can be affected by diet down to almost unmeasurable levels, you may still find that the total cholesterol level in your blood is unacceptably high. (Incidentally, *unacceptably high* is a subjective term, one that will be redefined in the course of this chapter; suffice it to say that previously accepted norms are, in my opinion, "unacceptably high.")

Indeed, there are vast numbers of people who simply will not respond to nondrug therapy, and you really can't tell whether you fall into this category until you try. There are no markers based on your lifestyle, your diet, your weight, that can tell you whether your cholesterol level is too high or too low until you measure it.

For example, the person who runs eight miles a day and is thin as a rail and subsists primarily on a great high-fiber, low-cholesterol, low-fat diet can still have a dangerously high level of cholesterol in his blood. As an individual, you cannot look in the mirror and say, "My God, I'm overweight and I just had a bagel with extra cream cheese; therefore, my cholesterol must be high." Nor can you say, "I'm five-feet-ten-inches, 155 pounds, and eat well, so I must be safe." It sounds logical, but it's not.

Does that mean there aren't connections between lifestyle and heart disease? Of course not. Obesity and heart disease often go hand in hand. As do fitness and lower risks of heart disease. But we're talking specifically here about cholesterol. The only way to really know for sure where you stand is to have your cholesterol level checked. There is nothing that I can say that absolves you of the responsibility of checking your cholesterol level. In fact, I think it's the cornerstone of knowing the truth about your heart disease risk, and then dealing with it.

Although cholesterol is (obviously) as old as humankind, its leading role in the heart disease story wasn't recognized until the middle part of the twentieth century. The Framingham Study and other comprehensive, population-based studies looked closely at the amount of lipid in the blood of the human body. It made sense to look at the amount of lipid in the blood because autopsies had already demonstrated that plaque was filled with fatty substances, such as cholesterol-like compounds; it was only natural to wonder where that cholesterol came from. Yes, it wound up in the arteries, but it seemed unlikely that it had been manufactured in these arteries. Framingham and the other studies found that there was indeed a correlation between death of heart disease and the level of cholesterol in the blood. It was established statistically that people with a high serum cholesterol level were at increased risk for heart attack.

The more people looked at the biological mechanisms of cholesterol, the more complicated it appeared to be. For example,
we found high-density lipoprotein (HDL) and low-density li-
porotein (LDL) formed part of your total cholesterol number.
And we quickly discovered that HDL was good and LDL was
bad—you wanted more of the good cholesterol in your body and
less of the bad cholesterol.

Doctors focused more on the LDL, and the numbers they
wanted to see, but in fact the best advice is simply to get your
total cholesterol level down. If you want to fractionate it, fine.
The bang for your buck is in reducing your LDL level. But if you
lower the overall cholesterol level, the overwhelming likelihood
is that LDL level is going down, and you'll be in better shape
and less likely to have heart disease.

That leads to another important question, one whose answer
has been massaged and altered many times over the last half-
century:

What is an appropriate level of cholesterol?

No one has ever offered a definitive answer. There were assumptions carried throughout the 1960s, 1970s, and 1980s that
lower was better than higher, and that doctors should focus their
efforts on patients with extremely high levels of cholesterol. The
rationale was twofold: first, these patients were in the greatest
danger; second, it was easier to obtain dramatic results with
these patients—after all, they had further to fall. This was all
part of the "who is at the highest risk" approach to heart disease. Focus on the patients seemingly in the greatest danger,
and let everyone else fend for himself.

When we began to look at cholesterol levels and people's
risk of dying of heart disease, we found that the American population could be stratified into three groups: high-risk, moderate-
risk, low-risk. (Nobody is at no risk, by the way.) I think it was a

reasonable decision for doctors to focus on those at greatest risk because they were in closest proximity to death. Early cholesterol studies focused on people with very high cholesterol levels, and it was discovered that lifestyle factors—diet modification, weight reduction, and exercise—seemed to make the most difference in this group, not only because you could get more movement in their cholesterol, but because they were at high risk for dying anyway, and almost anything seemed to help. Even if their cholesterol level didn't change much, you could help them by modifying other risk factors. That is to say, if someone with a high cholesterol level quits smoking, that person is less likely to die, regardless of whether his cholesterol level moves a single point. So doctors naturally decided to concentrate on the most unhealthy group of people and decided to try to move them from high risk to moderate risk.

Again, this made sense. If you could get someone from a high-risk pool into a medium-risk pool, you had done a great service. If you could get that person to a low level of risk, well, you were pretty sure you had prolonged his life. For example, if you could get a patient to lower his cholesterol level from 300 to 220, you felt you'd earned your salary for the year. And rightfully so, because in the era before safe pharmacological intervention, it was almost impossible to achieve such results.

Not that we didn't try. In the late 1970s and 1980s, people went to extraordinary lengths, embracing diets that were, quite literally, fat-free or taking drugs that purported to remove dietary fat from the gastrointestinal tract before it was absorbed into the bloodstream. These were horrible drugs to ingest, because fat that isn't absorbed has to go somewhere. It doesn't just disappear. Inevitably, the desperate patients who tried these drugs suffered raging, fat-filled diarrhea and other gastrointestinal problems. Interestingly enough, a lot of people were willing to tolerate these unpleasant side effects, and a lot of doctors were only too happy to aid in their misery by prescribing the drugs. Why? Because, at the time, there was no better course of treatment, and for some of these patients, the only other option was death.

What was hidden in all of this—and I guess it comes under the rubric of "It's hard to remember while you're being attacked by alligators that you really came here to drain the swamp"— was the fact that few people focused on the standards that had been established. Everyone was looking at these high-risk folks and trying to get them down to so-called normal cholesterol levels of 210 and 220. Few people asked the million-dollar question: *Why do we think 220 is normal?* In the United States, for some reason, we have always considered the low 200s (adjusted for age, of course) to be a relatively safe and healthy level of cholesterol. As we've discovered, though, even those people with cholesterol level in the low 200s have been dying of heart attacks. Cardiovascular disease, in all its forms, remains the number one killer in America. Even if you remove that cohort of patients whose cholesterol level was astronomically high—people who consume a great deal of the interest in the medical community—the rate of death due to cardiovascular disease is quite high. So it's reasonable to ask, after all these years, *What is normal?* Why should a cholesterol level in the low 200s be considered normal if people with these numbers are still dying of heart attacks at alarming rates?

Part of the explanation is sociological. There are cultures in which "normal" cholesterol levels do seem to be lower. Historically, for example, Japanese eating a traditional diet low in cholesterol seem to have lower rates of heart disease. That's changed in recent years, of course, as the Japanese diet has been impacted by Western influence, with its emphasis on red meat and fast food. You could, in fact, look at three cohorts of

Japanese—those living in Japan, those living in Hawaii, and those living in the United States—and you would find that the "normal" cholesterol level would climb as you moved toward the United States. That's probably because the group in Japan is eating far more fish, a typical Japanese diet; the group in Hawaii is eating a mixed diet, Asian and Western; and the group in the continental United States is eating the junk that the rest of us in the West eat.

So, why hold Americans to such a dismal standard? A cholesterol level of 220? That's not a bad number to get down to if you've started with a level of 300 and have been moving heaven and Earth to knock that number down. But suppose you're starting at 220 or so? You're supposedly at "low risk," so you're not going to get much attention. You should, though, because there is an advantage to taking people whose cholesterol level is seemingly normal and reducing their cholesterol level even further—dramatically further. This is new and exciting information.

The data are collected in part from research focusing on people who had other risk factors for death due to heart disease: specifically diabetics. In other words, if the reason that people weren't looking in great depth at patients with so-called normal cholesterol level was that they were not dying as fast as the people in the high-risk group, then why not start looking at people dying of heart disease at astounding rates because they were at high risk for some other reason? When this shift was made, it became clear that diabetics with a cholesterol level of 220 were dying much faster than nondiabetics with a cholesterol level of 220. Then there was a series of studies that looked at dramatic drug intervention for diabetics whose cholesterol level fell into the so-called normal range, and when these people were given a class of drugs known as *statins* to lower their cholesterol level to approximately 180, the impact was impressive. As this particular group of patients was moved off the American norm and down toward lower levels of cholesterol, their death rate due to heart attack was reduced, and their incidence of heart attack per se was reduced.

That, naturally, led to another question: If diabetics do better with a cholesterol level well below 220, why not recommend a similar level for the rest of the United States? America is a nation that is dying of cholesterol poisoning. Our diet is high in cholesterol, our average cholesterol level is higher than the average in many other nations, and our heart attack rate is enormous.

It's possible that some groups in our heterogeneous society process dietary cholesterol poorly and have a genetic predisposition to high cholesterol levels and heart attack. Other groups may be more prone to diabetes, or high blood pressure and hence to heart disease.

It's not simply that all Americans eat too much cholesterol (and that may not be true either; check out the diet and exercise chapter); it's that the cholesterol we eat isn't processed precisely the same way by each of us. And in each of us, the cholesterol in our blood interacts with a complex and unique set of other associated risk factors. It's like saying, "Does eating sugar give you diabetes?" Well, no. Diabetics are intolerant of sugar and, without treatment they will have high sugar level in their blood. It follows, then, that diabetics should avoid exacerbating the situation by ingesting too much sugar. Similarly, people with a genetic predisposition to high cholesterol level should eat less cholesterol.

We have to make a distinction between "normal" and "healthy." *Normal* simply means "what everybody else is, statistically." When it comes to cholesterol and the American population, believe me, normal is not healthy. So, the answer to the question is we should reduce the American norm to somewhere in the vicinity of 180. That, in my estimation, is a far more acceptable number, and one that could save millions of lives. The problem is, without statins there is really no way to move the population off the current American norm. Sorry, diet doctors and exercise gurus, but that's the plain and simple truth. Much of your advice is sound and practical, but it's insufficient to achieve the dramatic results I'm proposing. We need more help. We need statins.

So, what are statins? You've seen the advertisements; you've heard the glowing recommendations and the warnings. But what are they? Statins are, simply, chemicals that occur in nature, chemicals that, when ingested, turn off part of the body's cholesterol-manufacturing process. There is a complicated chemical cascade of steps that the body uses in the production of cholesterol, and statins quite effectively interrupt some of the steps in this process. As a result, although the liver wants to make cholesterol, it can't. If you want a visual aid, then think of a wall of dominoes, lined up, ready to fall neatly. Each domino represents a step in the cholesterol manufacturing process. Each domino, or chemical step, needs the one behind it to fall first, then knock it over, so that it can in turn tip over the next domino. The dominoes must be lined up perfectly. Remove a single domino and the chain reaction stops—immediately! Statins modulate the cholesterol factory by removing one or more dominoes from the chain. The liver doesn't stop producing cholesterol completely, of course—that would be catastrophic— but it produces smaller amounts (how small depends on the dosage of the drug administered). The liver also gets selfish and holds on to more and more of the cholesterol molecules instead of releasing them into the blood. The net result is a dramatic drop in the cholesterol level in the blood.

Used wisely, statins give us a tremendous amount of power over our own health. Remember, diet and exercise are responsible for approximately 20 percent of your cholesterol level; your liver controls the other 80 percent. Therefore, even people who are at comparatively low risk can benefit from statins. You don't have to have a cholesterol level of 300 to see results. If your cholesterol level is 220, even 200 or 180, and you take statins, your cholesterol level will drop. No question about it. And the latest research shows that your risk of heart attack will decrease, too. That's the bottom line.

The story of statins is fascinating. It begins with a Japanese researcher named Akira Endo. He suspected that in the plant world there are molds that create chemicals that interfere with cholesterol production. This would be a mold's defense mechanism against other organisms that want to attack the mold. Some bacteria that attack mold (yes it's pretty dangerous in the mold world; bacteria are out to get you all the time) apparently need cholesterol to live, so a cholesterol-blocking compound would be bacteria-unfriendly. After testing more than 6,000 different candidate molds (and spending two years in the search), Dr. Endo found one that secretes a chemical that turns off a bacteria's ability to make cholesterol, thereby keeping the mold-world safe from the scourge of mold-eating bacteria.

If that sounds complicated, it is. If it sounds as if searching for drugs this way is a brand-new idea, it's not. The discovery of statins is similar to the discovery of another famous drug. More than fifty years ago Dr. Alexander Fleming found a mold that secretes a chemical; the chemical, in turn, defends the mold against bacteria. Dr. Fleming had found penicillin. Dr. Endo was following in Dr. Fleming's footsteps. And the drug Dr. Endo found, mevastatin, is as important as Dr. Fleming's. Even more fascinating, the mold Dr. Endo used was a close relative of the one Dr. Fleming studied, a member of the Penicillium family.

Later, two American physicians, Michael S. Brown and Joseph L. Goldstein, demonstrated that statins could dramatically lower LDL cholesterol in blood. In an elegant series of experiments they showed how interfering with the "domino" cascade alters the way the liver stores and releases the stuff. They won the Nobel Prize for their work in 1985.

Since that time, pharmaceutical companies have followed one of two paths in the creation and marketing of statins: Some are created directly from fungi—those are the so-called natural statins—and the others are synthetic modifications produced in the test tube. Practically speaking, natural and synthetic statins are virtually indistinguishable. They both perform the same function: They modulate the body's cholesterol factory and do so remarkably well.

As of this writing, there are six types of statins: atorvastatin, cerivastatin, fluvastatin, lovastatin, pravastatin, and simvastatin. All of these drugs, available commercially, perform the same basic function: They inhibit the body's endogenous cholesterol production, meaning the body's production of cholesterol, as opposed to the dietary contribution of cholesterol. Are they interchangeable? Not quite. For example, statistically, the statins that produce the greatest percentage of change in LDL cholesterol are atorvastatin and simvastatin. The most cost-effective statins are fluvastatin and atorvastatin. Given that information, you don't have to be a genius to figure out that atorvastatin seems to be the best drug on the market at this time. It's relatively inexpensive, extremely powerful, and easily tolerated. In terms of "cost per year of life saved" (a favorite term of insurance companies everywhere), atorvastatin is a real good actor. So, if I had to pick a single statin available on the market right now as the one to beat, atorvastatin would be it.

Still, there isn't a great deal of difference within the group. All of these are basically the same drug; they're just different variations on a theme. A statin by any other name would still lower your cholesterol and improve your lipid profile. Also, I have no preference for natural or synthetic. In fact, there are several synthetic statins in clinical trials right now, and some of them appear to be even more powerful and cost-effective than the current crop. That's typical of the pattern of the American pharmaceutical industry, especially when there is so much competition among various manufacturers. Over time, the drugs get more powerful, the consumer gets more choices, and the drugs go down in price. Eventually, as the patents run out, we get generic forms of these drugs, which cause prices to plummet. The important point to keep in mind is this: The statins we have on the market today are so effective, and have so few side effects, that even if there is a new superstatin out there somewhere, you should be able to use one of the ones we already have and call it a day.

With that in mind, let's talk a little bit about cost. Statins aren't cheap, but they aren't hugely expensive either. Estimated costs range from $1.29 per day (for a 20-milligram dose) for fluvastatin to as much $7.50 for lovastatin. This becomes yet another discussion of risk/benefit ratio. You can analyze the case for statins on an individual, patient-by-patient basis. Or you can ask whether paying for statins for more people saves society money in the long run. Statins make sense for society. They make sense for individuals as well. Cost will have to be addressed sooner rather than later. As we'll see, the insurance companies may be able to help out here.

The medical and scientific communities have investigated the efficacy and safety of statins with enormous vigor. The first studies were done on patients at very high risk for heart attack with a high cholesterol level—maybe they'd already suffered their first heart attack. And the results were overwhelming: Statins lowered cholesterol level and saved lives, no question about it. The next studies involved patients who had high cholesterol level but no past history of heart disease. Here, too, cholesterol level went down and the death rate improved. Then the studies progressed to patients with other high-risk factors, such as lifestyle and weight. In these people, too, statins proved to have lifesaving capabilities. Finally, today, we're seeing the most interesting study—and it's still under way—one that examines low-risk patients with a normal lipid profile. What we're seeing is that even this group, when treated with statins, has significantly fewer heart attacks.

One intriguing aspect of this study is that the death rate, the actual rate at which people with "normal" cholesterol level keeled over, compared to the death rate of controls (people with normal cholesterol level who didn't take statins) was only marginally different. The group who took statins had fewer heart attacks, but the death rates of the two groups were virtually the same. So the question is, Can you recommend statins for this group even though they don't seem to be dying all that fast? In my view the obvious answer is, Absolutely! The reason is straightforward: Wouldn't you rather *not* have a heart attack?

Regardless of whether the death rate in this group changes, any heart attack is a potential death experience. If you told me there was a drug that would prevent me from having a heart attack, would I take it? Of course I would. Whether the death rate is different is irrelevant to me. I don't care whether statistically a heart attack is unlikely to kill me; a heart attack is a bad thing to have. I know. I've seen enough of them.

It may turn out that the death rate will be lower for the statin-treated normal cholesterol level group. The study is still going on. Since this group will have fewer heart attacks than the high-risk group, it's going to take longer to get a statistically significant sample for their heart attack risk.

Let's talk for a moment about numbers. If you've read this far, you're probably wondering what I'm going to recommend in terms of statin therapy. Is there a specific number, a line of demarcation, separating those who should take statins from those who shouldn't? Not really.

The question is not, What is the ideal cholesterol level? The question is, Who should be on these drugs? And the answer is, Virtually everybody. In other words, it doesn't really matter whether I have a specific ideal number for your cholesterol level. I'm telling you that people who have a "normal" cholesterol level who take statins still get increased protection against heart attacks.

As with all medical therapy, there is a point of diminishing returns. But that's why the study on so-called normals is so impressive. It demonstrates that although there may be diminishing returns, there are returns nonetheless. If statin risks are low, then the risk/benefit ratio favors taking the pills.

For the past few years, doctors have been taking a look at LDL cholesterol levels in regard to overall risks, and they've been willing to say that if you're a high-risk person, your LDL cholesterol level should be no higher than 100; if you're a low-risk person, it should be below 130. To me, that makes no sense at all, specifically in light of the most recent studies on healthy people with a normal cholesterol level, in which heart attack risk was reduced by as much as 30 percent. It seems asinine to me that just because you're low risk, you should have to tolerate an LDL level of 130.

Recent research suggests that there is *no* level of LDL cholesterol below which we stop seeing a heart attack prevention advantage. This is called the absence of a threshold *effect*. Lower LDL cholesterol level correlates with lower heart attack risk—period. The most recent papers suggest that we shoot for an LDL cholesterol level of 80 or below if we want to maximize their benefits!

The least you can expect from a cholesterol-lowering statin, even if you're in the low-risk category, is that you'll be much less likely to have a heart attack. You'll be less likely to experience the joy of chest pain, a visit to the emergency room, followed by a trip to the coronary care unit and an angioplasty. Even in this group, statins have been shown to reduce heart attack risk by 30 percent. Thirty percent! With that kind of evidence, I think it's a sin that statins aren't more readily available to the American public.

If you'd like an odd and rather subtle marker to attest to what I've been telling you, look no further than your friendly local medical insurance company or your health maintenance organization (HMO). They have begun, quietly, and without much fanfare, to pay for statins even for people with so-called normal lipid profiles. Insurance executives are not the most altruistic folks in the world. They look at public health in economic terms. They evaluate life and death issues in terms of cold hard cash. What do they know, or believe, that the FDA and the rest of the medical establishment are unwilling to tell you? Might it be that it's cheaper, in the long run, to pay a few hundred dollars a year for statins than to get stuck with a $50,000 bill for a coronary care admission down the line? I can't tell you for sure. I'm not invited to insurance company boardrooms all that often (come to think of it, I'm *never* invited). But it should give you pause. It seems to me that the insurance folks are telling you exactly the same thing that I am, with a little nudge and a wink.

To me, this one is a no-brainer. By taking these relatively inexpensive drugs, you can prevent relatively expensive complications. For the high-risk people—people who have had a heart attack, whose cholesterol level is 300—no one is arguing. These people absolutely have to be on statins. The issue becomes increasingly fuzzy as you begin to talk about people whose situation isn't quite so grave. The healthier you are, the lower your cholesterol level, the more likely you are to run into opposition.

That's backward. Given the data we have so far—the drug companies have shown these drugs work, but more importantly, the data show they save lives and at the very least prevent people from getting very sick (because there is no way to define a heart attack as anything other than being very sick)—it seems to me that anyone who is charged with contributing to the health care of America—whether it be a doctor, a nurse, a health-reimbursement company, or an insurance company—should be in favor of this treatment. This is a simple, inexpensive, straightforward, well-tolerated therapy, one that every insurance company has an ethical, moral, incontrovertible duty to reimburse.

This advice will surely seem extreme to some observers, though I don't know why. In the years before statins, people were willing to go to enormous lengths to lower their cholesterol level and maintain their fitness and overall cardiovascular health. Now we've made it easier. We've made it as simple as taking a pill. Is that such a terrible thing? At the risk of sounding like an idealist, should we deny anyone the advantages of a lower cholesterol level just because it's achieved by taking a pill that costs somebody some money? There are hidden costs in everything. How much do running shoes cost you per year? Your tennis racket? Your golf clubs? How expensive is the risk of being hit by a car while you're jogging down the street, fighting the good fight, trying to stay fit?

If you want to make sure that your doctor will prescribe a statin for you, just embrace a bad habit. Get fat, start smoking, raise your blood pressure. Become desperately ill. You'll get your statins. This way lies madness!

Why should you be discriminated against because you're doing everything right?

This antiquated, wasteful, immoral approach to health care will change only if people demand that it change. The general public will have to insist that their heart health will be protected. This is not unprecedented. Women have fought for, and received, the right to have experimental, expensive, high-risk breast cancer therapy included in their health care plans—specifically, bone marrow transplants. In reality, there wasn't a lot of good evidence that bone marrow transplant increases the survival rate tremendously, and yet the courts ruled that because people demanded it, the insurance companies must reimburse for it.

With statins, we have documented evidence, excellent science and voluminous studies, that statins reduce the incidence of heart attack for virtually anyone, regardless of level of risk. With this kind of proof at hand, I don't understand why doctors don't prescribe, and why some insurance company holdouts don't reimburse for, statin therapy in low-risk patients.

A final note on the benefits of statins. They have more than one activity. The first assumption about statins was that they reduced the risk of heart disease by reducing the amount of cholesterol in the blood. The LDL level went down, and as a result the amount of fat in the wall of the artery was reduced; subsequently, the amount of inflammation went down, and as a result, you were at less risk of having a heart attack. But there is new evidence suggesting that this effect may not be the only benefit of statins. They may have a direct anti-inflammatory effect as well. If you give statins to people with high levels of C-reactive protein, the C-reactive protein level comes down faster than you would expect if the statins were just doing this indirectly by reducing the fat level in the blood. So statins may have the added benefit of complementing the anti-inflammatory effect of aspirin.

Enthusiastic as my endorsement of statins may be, it does include a few caveats. Although statins have been shown to be extremely safe and effective, they are powerful drugs and as such must be administered with a degree of care. Some statins are metabolized by the liver's cytochrome P450 enzyme pathway. Other drugs are metabolized by the same mechanism, so the potential for interaction with other drugs is a concern. This relationship will affect the dosage of each that you should take.

Similarly, drugs that are protein-bound (ask your doctor about the specific drugs you are taking) will compete with some statins for space in the bloodstream. Again, you may have to adjust some drug dosages. One of the classic interactions is between a statin and Coumadin, the anticoagulant taken by many heart patients. Therefore, it's very important to let your doctor know every drug you are taking before you begin statin therapy.

In addition, the cost of these drugs varies widely, and you may have to pay for them out of pocket. So there are some tricks you can try to make statins less expensive for you. If you need 20 milligrams of a statin, you can ask your doctor to prescribe the often less expensive 40-milligram pill, rather than the 20-milligram pill. (Don't ask why 40-milligram pills are cheaper. Apparently it's a drug company thing and we wouldn't understand.) Then you just cut the pill in half. That's an old doctor's trick that can significantly reduce cost.

Another trick is to combine the statin with grapefruit juice, which has the unique effect of increasing the blood level of some of these drugs dramatically (as much as nine times!) and therefore allows you to use half the dosage or less. Again, though, it's vital to communicate with your doctor on these matters. Some pills can't be cut. Grapefruit juice may be too unpredictable for your health situation.

The bottom line on statins is that they are truly miraculous drugs. Before statins we had the ability to wiggle your blood lipid level maybe 10 percent. Statins do that without even taking a deep breath. With statin therapy we can affect your blood lipid level by 30 percent or so, perhaps even more. Virtually every statin is going to be able to do that, regardless of what other modifications you make to your lifestyle.

Moreover, the tolerability and the safety of statins are unmatched by those of any of the cholesterol-lowering drugs currently or previously available. Statins are better tolerated in the sense that people are able to stay on them and feel good while they are on them. For example, studies show that about 96 percent of the people who begin statin therapy are able to keep taking the drugs for at least one year. Compare that to, say, niacin, another popular drug that has been used to combat high cholesterol level. Fewer than half of the people who take niacin are able to continue therapy for a year. Or consider the class of drugs known as *bile-acid sequestrants*, which were widely prescribed and considered quite safe. Unfortunately, people hated them, and only 35 percent were able to take them for a full year.

Admittedly, it's very hard to compare all drugs in all people, but there is no question that if you can get a 96 percent tolerability level with a new drug, you've got an all-star performer. Niacin wasn't a disaster, and there are doctors who still prescribe it today. Compared to statins, though, it's a minor league drug.

The truth is, almost any drug, any therapy, will have a lower tolerability rate than 96 percent. You could recommend a daily dosage of prune juice (for whatever reason), and you'd likely find less than 96 percent of the population could tolerate it for a full year. Statins are almost the perfect combination of effectiveness on one side and lack of toxicity on the other side. Think about it: 96 percent of all people tolerate statins so well that there is no reason to go off them. That is not to say that the drugs can't produce side effects. They can. Typically, they can produce some muscle pain, some alterations in the enzymes in your liver (which a blood test will determine), but for the vast majority of people taking these drugs, the side effects either end or never occur. We will discuss the public health implications at these effects later in chapter 12. The benefits, in my opinion, far outweigh the risks.

Statins have changed the landscape of treating heart disease. You can divide all of cardiology, all of medicine, into two eras: the era before statins and the era after statins. The only problems now are getting enough doctors to understand how good statins are and getting the creaky old medical bureaucracy to understand that it isn't just the gravely ill, the irresponsible, and the unfortunate who are candidates for statin therapy.

I'm a candidate.

And so are you.

CHAPTER SIX

Antibiotics

Some heart attacks may be caused by bacteria. That simple, straightforward sentence has provoked a storm of controversy during the past few years. There are still plenty of doctors who don't believe it, though their number is shrinking daily. Most of the public has never heard about the infectious disease–heart attack connection. But it's real. And it's exciting. Because if bacteria play a role in heart attacks, we can prevent heart attacks by giving people antibiotics.

If I had spoken to you a generation ago and told you that stomach ulcers were caused by infectious disease, you almost certainly would have laughed me out of the room. You might have said, "Oh, come on, Doc; ulcers are caused by stress and bad food. What you really need to fight ulcers are a good antacid and a less demanding job—or at least a vacation in the Bahamas." In response, I might well have shrugged my shoulders and slunk away, too uncertain of my evidence to put up much of a fight. Not anymore. What we know now is that ulcers are caused by infectious disease, specifically by bacteria known as

H. pylori. There is no dispute about this anymore. The bacteria lead ultimately to an irritation of the stomach, which in turn is exacerbated by stress, spicy food, and other lifestyle factors. In other words, what we thought we knew just a few short years ago was completely and utterly wrong.

That led to the obvious question: Are there other, similarly enigmatic ailments out there, conditions that may in fact be caused by bacteria, even though they appear to be diseases that don't have anything at all to do with infection? It appears now that the answer to that question is yes. Heart disease is one of them.

There have been rumblings about infection and heart disease for much longer than you might expect. Much of the research has gone on at the edges of mainstream cardiology. But only recently has anyone thought to put any serious effort into proving a causal relationship. Some eighty years ago it was suggested that the sclerosis of old age may simply be a summation of lesions arising from infectious or metabolic toxins. But we can go back even further, to 1852, when Dr. Carl Von Rokitansky tried to draw a link between infectious disease and something called "incrustation" of the heart. Four years later, in 1856, Dr. Rudolf Virchow came up with a hypothesis that plaque formation caused by lipids may be related to infection. In 1891, a Dr. Hutchard speculated that infectious disease in childhood may be related to heart disease later in life. And a Dr. Weisel postulated that heart disease could be caused by any number of infectious diseases, including typhoid fever, scarlet fever, and measles. The real heavy hitter, though, was the revered Canadian doctor William Osler, who in the early 1900s published his thoughts on the matter. They boiled down to this simple hypothesis: Acute infections are a cause of plaque in the arteries.

Since Osler was one of the great minds in the history of medicine, his imprimatur on this matter gave it considerable weight and naturally led others to follow his lead. There have been scores of papers published on this subject, and a mountain of research investigating the link between heart disease and any number of infectious diseases. But it was not until the 1980s that researchers suggested that infection causes an injury to the arterial wall, and the response of the body to the infection leads to inflammation and causes heart disease.

Why has it taken so long to make this connection? Because heart disease has always been a maddeningly complicated killer, one seemingly influenced by a host of factors. It wasn't until the late 1980s that scientists began to find real evidence of an infectious component of heart disease, and most of their research focused on a single, ubiquitous infection: chlamydia.

The first reports of a *Chlamydia* species in heart disease revolved around cases of infection inside the heart itself, not in the arteries. These reports were associated with the *Chlamydia* species more commonly found in gynecologic disease and reproductive disease, but there is another species of *Chlamydia* out there, something called *Chlamydia pneumoniae*, and when scientists began honing in on this species of *Chlamydia*, and its possible connection to cardiovascular disease, they hit pay dirt.

It's important to understand that there are many different strains of *Chlamydia*. *Chlamydia pneumoniae* is not a sexually transmitted disease. Most people assume all *Chlamydia* are alike, but they're not. There is the sexually transmitted *Chlamydia* infection, which affects the reproductive organs. And there is the *Chlamydia* infection caused by *Chlamydia pneumoniae*, which is not sexually transmitted. *C. pneumoniae* infects the lungs. And chlamydia pneumonia is everywhere.

Research has shown that worldwide the prevalence of antibodies against this bacterium approaches 50 percent. Fifty percent!

That means precisely what you think it means: that approximately half the people on the planet have been exposed to chlamydia pneumonia. (Incidentally, the figure runs about 25 percent higher in men than in women, and that is important, because we know that more men than women get heart attacks.) The majority of these cases are subclinical—meaning there are no symptoms, and you don't know you have them.

What exactly is chlamydia pneumonia? It's a respiratory disease exchanged most commonly through droplet infection: you breathe it in, just as in the common cold or flu or a host of other infections. It sounds harmless enough, right? I mean, how bad can it be if you don't even know you have it? Well, the problem with chlamydia pneumonia is not that it makes you feel terrible (as flu does), but that it has the potential to do far greater damage in other parts of your body. Worse, you probably won't even know it's happening—until too late!

The first study on this subject to gain worldwide attention was completed in Japan in 1988. In that study, scientists investigated a possible association between chlamydia pneumonia and coronary artery disease. They took blood samples from forty men who had experienced heart attacks, thirty men with demonstrated chronic coronary artery disease, and forty-one men in a control group, and they analyzed the samples for antibodies to *Chlamydia*. A whopping 68 percent of the patients who had suffered heart attacks, and 50 percent of the men with chronic coronary disease, showed elevated level of antibodies to *Chlamydia pneumoniae*. That was significantly higher than the percentage of the control group. The finding suggested that chronic chlamydia pneumonia infections might play a role in acute and chronic coronary disease. That was the first big bang, but there was more. When they looked more closely at this information, the research team found not only that these patients had antibodies to *Chlamydia*, but that just before their heart attack, or around the time of their heart attack, the number of antibodies increased dramatically.

So this is what they knew: People who suffered heart attacks had *Chlamydia* more often than the population at large. And many of these patients exhibited increased antibody activity right around the time of their heart attack, suggesting one of two things: either they were reinfected with *Chlamydia pneumoniae*, or the infection had never ended. It had simply lingered in the body, then flared just before the heart attack. This study, too, asked more questions than it answered, but at least it pushed the conversation in the right direction: toward a specific infectious disease, namely chlamydia pneumonia.

One of the many odd and fascinating characteristics of *Chlamydia pneumoniae* is that it is a bacterium whose presence in the body is made more hospitable by cigarette smoke. Simply put, you're more likely to have chronic *Chlamydia pneumoniae* infection if you are a smoker. This, of course, is a correlation that absolutely jumps off the page because it's related to a question that physicians and scientists have been asking for decades: Why is smoking associated with heart attack? No one ever had an answer. Oh, people had suggestions and ideas and possible connections, some more reasonable than others, but they never really had a solid answer.

"There's bad stuff in the smoke," they'd say, "radioactive compounds that affect the arteries."

Maybe. Maybe not.

"Smoking causes an increase in the amount of carbon monoxide in the blood, and that hurts your heart in the long run."

Okay. Sounds plausible.

Then again, maybe not.

The fact is, nobody could point directly to something in cigarettes, some particular substance or chemical compound, and
state, beyond a reasonable doubt, and backed by scientific evidence, "This is why cigarettes and heart attack are related." But
if we throw *Chlamydia pneumoniae* into the mix, then we have a
different equation.

People who are chronic smokers do damage to their lungs,
presumably because of the toxic material in the smoke. What we
now know, however, is that chromic smokers are also great hosts
for *Chlamydia pneumoniae* because *Chlamydia pneumoniae*
bacteria simply love to live in patients who have lungs damaged
by smoking. Moreover, if there are *Chlamydia pneumoniae* in
your lungs, there are probably *Chlamydia pneumoniae* in other
places as well. This realization led scientists to examine
Chlamydia pneumoniae much more closely. They began to wonder whether it might be directly linked to coronary artery disease and heart attack. In other words, they asked the question
that scientists had been asking for more than a century: Could
heart attack be an infectious disease, at least in part?

To answer this question with any degree of certainty and sat-
isfaction, scientists have routinely turned to a set of guidelines
known as *Koch's postulates*. Dr. Robert Koch was a brilliant German scientist who in the late nineteenth century devised a set of
conditions that must be met in order to prove that a disease is
caused by an infectious agent, and that the specific agent you
are looking at is the cause of the disease. These conditions,
which came to be known as *Koch's postulates*, are paraphrased
as follows:

1. *The agent has to be present in nearly all cases of the
   disease.* (This makes sense. For example, if the
   tuberculosis [TB] bacterium causes the symptoms of

tuberculosis, then the TB bacterium should be found in everyone who has the disease.)

2. *The agent must be isolated from someone who has the disease and then successfully cultivated in the laboratory.* (In this case, *Chlamydia pneumoniae* bacteria would be harvested from someone who had suffered a heart attack; then they would be grown in a laboratory environment.)

3. *The laboratory bacterium must be introduced to a host who does not yet have the disease and cause the disease in the new host.* (In the case of heart disease, the laboratory *Chlamydia pneumoniae* would be injected into someone who doesn't yet have heart disease. Then, if the process works as it should, heart disease would develop.)

4. *The new strain of bacterium must be retrieved from the new host and compared to the original strain.* If the two organisms match, then the circle is closed, and the pathogen is determined to cause the infectious disease you are studying. Said another way, the disease you are studying is caused by the specific infectious agent you have identified.

There is one serious problem with using Koch's postulates to prove that heart disease is an infectious disease: You have to kill someone to do it. Koch's postulates have been used countless times on nonlethal diseases. Heart attacks, unfortunately, are often lethal, so we'll have to modify the postulates a little. I realize that won't completely satisfy some purists, but I'm sure they'll understand that there is no way you can, of your own volition, satisfy Koch's postulates and prove that in humans, heart attacks are caused by chlamydial infections.

However:

You can apply Koch's postulates to animal studies. And in animals, guess what? They work! You can take animals, you can give them *Chlamydia pneumoniae*, and you'll discover that even animals without a lot of lipid in their diet get heart attacks. Then you can recover the *Chlamydia* bacteria from the animals that had heart attacks and close the circle. So, at least in animals—which may be the best evidence we will ever get, in terms of Koch's postulates—there is direct, dramatic scientific evidence that *Chlamydia pneumoniae* is in a very strong way a causal agent for heart attack.

We can go even further. What happens if we treat animals with antibiotics? It turns out that we can reduce their heart attack rate. So Koch's postulates, which were written before the era of antibiotics, can be extended to a fifth postulate, which is this: *If you give an antibiotic, or an agent, known to kill the punitive, causative agent of this disease, and you prevent the disease by giving this agent, that is added evidence that this agent is the cause of the illness.*

Therefore, we have here, at least in an animal model, the fulfillment of Koch's postulates. Now, in people, what do we have? We can fulfill the first of them. We are finding the agent, *Chlamydia*, in many people with obvious heart disease. It is unlikely that we will ever find the actual bacteria in *everybody* with the disease, simply because we don't often go in and invade these people's coronary arteries and suck it out, because that's dangerous. We can grow the recovered *Chlamydia* in the lab, but here the Koch's postulate circle must break down. We will never be able to introduce *Chlamydia* into healthy people and then watch to see whether they get heart attacks. So we have to get creative and look for other evidence.

We do have suggestive evidence that many people who have

suffered heart attacks are infected with *Chlamydia pneumoniae*. Remember, we already know that the disease is present in more than 50 percent of the population. Moreover, as you grow older, the more likely it is that you have *Chlamydia pneumoniae*. If we limit the demographic to people in their late sixties and seventies, we find that approximately 75 percent of them have antibodies to *Chlamydia pneumoniae*. Three-quarters of the population in that age bracket have, at some time in their life, acquired *Chlamydia pneumoniae*!

There's more, something quite subtle, that this statistic reveals. Once you've been infected and have recovered, your antibodies to *Chlamydia pneumoniae* should fade. The fact that the number of people who have antibodies actually *grows* over time suggests that people are constantly being reinfected with this disease. In order for the number of people with positive antibodies to *Chlamydia pneumoniae* to increase with age, the number of *Chlamydia* infections must be *enormous*. And it is, in fact, we're talking about an epidemic.

Numerous major studies have sought to demonstrate a link between *Chlamydia pneumoniae* and coronary artery disease— more than two dozen between 1988 and 1999 alone; of those, only four had a negative result. All of the others had positive results. These were not small, insignificant studies conducted at backwater research facilities. These were big, expensive studies performed under the umbrella of highly reputable institutions. Among the specific evidence: a 1992 study in which scientists examined microscopic pictures of plaque samples taken at autopsy from seven people known to have suffered from coronary artery disease. It appeared, at first glance, as though there were cellular particles within the plaque that resembled *Chlamydia pneumoniae*. Further tests confirmed the scientists' suspicions in five of the seven cases. Not only that, but a subsequent study, of ninety living patients who had undergone atherectomy (the removal of plaque from the coronary arteries), revealed that 79 percent tested positive for *Chlamydia pneumoniae*. Think about that. In this study, nearly eight of ten patients with coronary artery disease were also infected with *Chlamydia pneumoniae*. That's pretty powerful evidence.

In January 2000, an article in the *Medical Clinics of North America* asked a simple but profoundly important question related to heart disease and the possibility of a *Chlamydia* link: Why do so many people who don't have a lot of the commonly recognized risk factors for heart attack—diabetes, hypertension, high cholesterol level, tobacco use, family history—still have heart attacks? "These risk factors," the article stated, "combine to account for only about fifty percent of observed incidents of atherosclerosis. And they are only associations. The mechanism by which they contribute to the development of atherosclerosis is unclear." So, not only do we have 50 percent of the people without these risk factors, we don't really understand why these risk factors are risk factors! As we've begun to realize, many of these risk factors are also risk factors for *Chlamydia pneumoniae*. Surely that's not merely a coincidence.

A study conducted in Finland in 1999 focused on possible risk factors of coronary heart disease that have an effect on *Chlamydia* and the development of chronic infection. Put another way, there are certain factors that we know put you at high risk for heart disease; do they also put you at high risk for *Chlamydia pneumoniae*? The answer is yes: age, male gender, smoking. Additionally, it turns out that *Chlamydia* likes iron. If you have a diet high in iron, and your body has high iron stores, you are more likely to have *Chlamydia pneumoniae*. There is also evidence that if your body has high iron stores, you're more likely to have a heart attack. Stress, too, is a factor. People under great stress seem to be at higher risk of having *Chlamydia pneumoniae*, just as they are at higher risk of having a heart attack.

Now, going the other way, what are the risk factors for coronary heart disease that *Chlamydia pneumoniae* changes? If you have *Chlamydia pneumoniae*, that increases your chances of having chronic bronchitis, and we know people who have this condition are at increased risk of heart attack. If you have active *Chlamydia pneumoniae*, you will probably have elevated levels of C-reactive protein, and we know that people with an elevated C-reactive protein level have high heart attack rates. *Chlamydia pneumoniae* infection will raise cholesterol levels, all by itself. That, too, is a risk for heart attack. Infection with *Chlamydia pneumoniae* will lower the level of HDL cholesterol—another risk factor. We also know that people with *Chlamydia* are often overweight, and that is another risk factor for heart disease.

It's amazing, really, how many of these perplexing aspects of the heart disease risk picture—*Why should X, Y, Z make you at risk for heart disease?*—make sense if you realize that *Chlamydia pneumoniae* produce the same phenomena, and they're showing up on the statistical studies as heart disease risks. They're actually the effects of *Chlamydia pneumoniae*! Flip it around yet again: *Why are these heart disease risks? Because some of them place you at high risk for* Chlamydia. This may not be Koch's postulates at work; nevertheless, we're seeing powerful evidence that something is going on with *Chlamydia* in the heart attack mix.

Here's another example, a study in which eleven rabbits were fed a normal diet, then given *Chlamydia pneumoniae* intranasally. Within four weeks, two of the rabbits developed heart disease. In a separate study, rabbits were infected with *Chlamy-*

dia pneumoniae. Some were given antibiotics and others were not. Then the rabbits were fed diets rich in cholesterol. The result? A significant acceleration of plaque formation in the aorta of infected rabbits when compared to rabbits whose *Chlamydia pneumoniae* had been treated.

Admittedly, this is all relatively new information, especially when measured against the clock of science and medicine, which too often moves at a snail's pace. Still, in my opinion, it's more than just a medical curiosity. It's strongly suggestive that, at the very least, there is an infectious disease component of coronary artery disease. This finding offers even greater support for the notion that the inflammatory response is one of the fundamental reasons why people die of heart attacks.

Are there other infectious diseases that could be culpable? Sure there are, but none of them fits quite as well. Scientists have looked closely at some viral infections, but the evidence is not as impressive. Chronic dental infections do seem to correlate to heart attack rates. In the dental infection case, a potential scenario goes something like this: The older you get the more likely you are to have chronic dental infections. People with chronic dental infections often get bacteria in their blood. Some of these bacteria find their way into the coronary arteries. The chronic inflammatory state in the gums is then associated with a chronic inflammatory state in the coronary arteries. Is the dental infection evidence overwhelming? No, the *Chlamydia* evidence is far stronger. But stay tuned. Developments are occurring rapidly in the infectious disease–heart attack field.

For now, the smart money is on *Chlamydia pneumoniae*. The synthesis of all this research on *Chlamydia pneumoniae* and heart disease can be boiled down to a handful of basic evidence:

1. If you look for antibodies to *Chlamydia pneumoniae* in the blood, you find them more often in people who have had heart attacks than in the general population.
2. An examination of arterial wall tissue from heart attack victims often reveals *Chlamydia pneumoniae*.
3. When animals are injected with *Chlamydia pneumoniae*, heart disease develops; moreover, when their chlamydial infection is treated, their incidence of heart disease is reduced.
4. Preliminary antichlamydial antibiotic studies, both in animals and in humans, seem to reduce the incidence of heart attack.
5. Chronic chlamydial infection produces chronic inflammation. That should increase C-reactive protein levels in the blood, just what we see in people at high risk for heart attack.

To me, those are five pretty strong reasons to believe that chlamydia pneumonia and heart disease are related. We can add to this list the rest of the incriminating evidence.

Chlamydia pneumoniae is a unique bug in that it likes to sit in the coronary arteries, and we haven't found a lot of other bugs in there. It's unique in that it's very easy to transmit. It's unique in that it affects 50 to 75 percent of the population, and significantly more men than women, more smokers than nonsmokers. In fact, the more you look at chlamydia pneumonia and the way it distributes itself in the American population, the more it resembles the distribution of heart disease: older people, more men than women, an association with smoking. Not only that, *Chlamydia pneumoniae* can affect people's lipid profile—it makes HDL level go down and LDL level go up. So this is a very bad-smelling organism. It just feels wrong to have it around.

The disease is so ubiquitous that it may not even make sense, in terms of public health, or even for you personally, to be tested for *Chlamydia pneumoniae*. So it is reasonable to say:

I don't need to be tested for Chlamydia. *I'll just assume I'm positive and get treated.* The older you are, the more likely that statement is to be true. The younger you are, the more benefit you should achieve from *Chlamydia* eradication. The only questions that remain, then, are related to risk/benefit ratio. There is a risk/benefit ratio of this program for individuals to assess, and another for society as a whole to consider.

For any given individual the risk of *Chlamydia* infection is relatively high. The risk of a brief course of antibiotics is quite low. For society, the question is slightly more complicated. The risk of untreated chlamydial infection among millions of people is an epidemic of heart attacks. That epidemic costs billions of dollars in medical expense, lost income, lost experience in the workplace, not to mention its toll in human misery. So treating *Chlamydia* can benefit all of us in a material way. The risk of the treatment would be the development of so-called superbugs, the antibiotic-resistant strains of bacteria that emerge when antibiotics are overused and distributed to millions of people without real justification. But a brief course of antibiotics should minimize the risk. And we might be able to develop a national policy of "rotating" antibiotics so that no single drug is overused. Both risk/benefit arguments, then, seem to converge on a simple recommendation: Get rid of the *Chlamydia pneumoniae* bacteria in your body if you can.

Does that mean everyone should be given a course of antibiotics without testing for chlamydial antibodies first? Sounds crazy on the surface, perhaps, but in fact, if you were to give an antibiotic to every adult in America, you'd be giving it to the wrong people only 25 percent of the time.

For how long should you be treated? Studies show a variety of responses to the question. Some scientists are recommending two weeks of treatment; others are recommending bursts of as little as one to three days. To me, anything in that range is acceptable for dealing with the issue of chlamydia pneumonia as it relates to heart disease.

If you'd like to monitor yourself after getting antibiotics and then see whether you reacquire antibodies to *Chlamydia*, that doesn't really sound crazy. Good luck finding a lab, though.

Am I telling you that part of this program involves walking into your doctor's office and asking for a course of antibiotics to rid your body of a possible chlamydial infection? Yes, that's what I'm telling you. Take control of your health. Believe it or not, your doctor will probably not put up much of a fight, especially if you're armed with the right information.

It would be necessary to make this a public health policy, with oversight, of course: We don't want to give people random antibiotics whenever they want them; we don't want to give them enormous quantities of broad-spectrum antibiotics at the drop of a hat; we don't want the American public to be continuously on antibiotics to the point that we get bacteria in our environment that are not responsive to antibiotics at any time.

But, if we have a specific target—in this case, *Chlamydia pneumoniae*, which affects an enormous percentage of the population—there is nothing wrong with giving a specific course of antibiotics for a specific self-limited period. I think if you were to poll the medical and scientific community, a significant number of its members, me among them, would say that this makes sense.

Remember, too, that a significant number of people won't have to be treated, because they've already been on antibiotics in the recent past; however, not all antibiotics are effective in the eradication of *Chlamydia* organisms.

One other group deserving special attention here are high-risk patients waiting for coronary bypass surgery, people with demonstrated coronary artery disease. These are people who are put on a waiting list until an operating room is available. They are at high risk of dying. So the question has been raised, in an ongoing study, whether certain antibiotics, most notably azythromyicin, might reduce the risk of complications in bypass surgery. Preliminary indications are that the answer is yes. So, if you're waiting for surgery, you might want to ask your doctor about that.

Here's something else to consider when assessing the relative risks and benefits associated with antibiotic therapy. Heart disease risk peaked in the late 1970s. Yes, it's still the number one killer in the United States, but it's not quite as high as it once was. If you were to graph the heart disease epidemic across time, the shape of this graph would resemble the shape of nothing so much as an infectious disease epidemic, which typically burns brightly and fiercely through a population and then slowly fades away. In addition, the gradual decrease in heart disease in this country parallels the increased use of antibiotics. That's right: The proliferation of antibiotics, which so many people have been decrying for the past twenty to thirty years, may have had at least one beneficial effect. There is, in fact, evidence to suggest that our wanton use of antibiotics, which has been so roundly (and appropriately) criticized as a risk for the production of superbugs, has in its own unexpected way contributed to the ablation of the heart disease risk in America. This is another example of Murphy's law of biology: *Sometimes things just happen.*

Give antibiotics to everyone!

That sounds so bad on the surface that many infectious disease specialists go berserk when you suggest it. But phrase it a different way and they feel better about it. We have an infectious epidemic of heart disease in this country. We should try to focus the antibiotic therapy, laserlike, on the most likely pathogen, which is *Chlamydia pneumoniae*. We should give it for the briefest possible time that we think will produce a clinically significant result and then stop. The fact that we got lucky in our research and reached this conclusion almost by accident is irrelevant. Why not use the information to save lives?

What is the mechanism behind the *Chlamydia pneumoniae*–heart attack connection? How does it actually cause disease? Once again, we go back to our old friend inflammation, and the inflammatory response.

STEP 1: Substrate exists in the coronary arteries that makes *Chlamydia* happy. That is, there's food for bacteria in the arteries, probably in some fatty substances there, either because the body has produced too much fat on its own or because for some reason *Chlamydia* infection actually produced in the body a fat profile that makes it easier for *Chlamydia* to live. (It's more likely the former than the latter, though if you're a bacterium and can force the body to make some extra food for you to eat, so much the better. As to why *Chlamydia* can do this at all, the best explanation I have to offer is simple Darwinian selection. All the other bacteria that couldn't perform this particular trick died. *Chlamydia* is all that's left. Not a very satisfying explanation, I admit, but it's all we've got right now.)

Either way, the *Chlamydia* find that living in a body in which there is lipid in the coronary artery makes them very happy. So they load up the U-Haul and move in. In so doing, they annoy the hell out of the body's immune system. (After all, the body's immune system is supposed to be annoyed by stuff like *Chlamydia* living in it, unbidden.)

STEP 2: Enter the immune response. Not because it's mysteriously attacking your coronary arteries out of the blue; not because cigarette smoke in some bizarre way cranks up the immune response, and it just so happens it attacks the coronary arteries; not even because you didn't exercise enough or your immune system got mad at you. The immune system responds for a purely logical reason: because there is a specific target in the coronary arteries that it is designed to attack. And it does, through inflammation. Then, because a chlamydial infection is present and isn't being eliminated, the inflammatory response smolders along, creating more debris, more matter that is injurious to the structure of the coronary artery walls.

STEP 3: After a while, because the inflammatory response hasn't been turned off, the debris begins to drill through the artery wall. When that happens—bang! Blood clot. Obstruction! Heart attack!

It is true that for every complicated problem there is a simple, straightforward solution that is easy to understand, inexpensive to implement, and *wrong!* But my program seems to be an exception to that rule. Every time you look, the evidence accumulates: *Chlamydia pneumoniae* is found in the arteries; *Chlamydia* antibodies are found in the blood. Factors that promote *Chlamydia pneumoniae* growth in the human body, such as tobacco smoke and lung damage, also promote heart attack. The incidence of *Chlamydia pneumoniae* increases with age, as does the incidence of heart attack. *Chlamydia pneumoniae* is more common in men than in women; same with heart attack. Animals infected with *Chlamydia pneumoniae* have heart attacks; animals treated against *Chlamydia pneumoniae* have fewer heart attacks. The heart attack incidence numbers resemble an infectious disease curve.

The evidence is overwhelming. If *Chlamydia* were on trial, and I heard the prosecuting attorney giving his summation, pointing at that *Chlamydia* bug, I would convict the bug and send it away.

CHAPTER SEVEN

Angina

Throughout the majority of this book we've honed in on the latest and greatest information available in the war against heart attack. The war against heart attack is a war against soft plaque.

But what about angina? Angina remains a significant problem in the United States (and indeed throughout the world). As with heart attack, angina is provoked by disease in the heart vessels, the coronary arteries; it causes tremendous disability and discomfort, and when it is severe, it is associated with an increased risk of death. But angina is caused by hard plaque, not soft plaque. So, you might reasonably ask, is there anything that our program—which has been demonstrated to be so effective in combating heart attacks—has to offer angina sufferers?

Yes.

If you have angina, you aren't left out of the mix. Certainly, you should go on this program because you don't want to have a heart attack—that's reason enough. But people with angina, those with hard plaque, have an increased risk for heart attack because one of the markers for soft plaque is hard plaque. Apart from that, is there anything that this program offers you, the longtime sufferer of angina, apart from decreasing your risk of death of heart attack? Again, the answer is, yes.

There are at least 16 million people in the United States who suffer from chronic angina, and that's a conservative estimate. Because angina is a disease that is often ignored or misdiagnosed in the early stages, many people endure the discomfort for some time without knowing its cause. Indeed, it's more likely that the number of Americans who have angina is closer to 20 million. That's about one out of every fifteen people. It is, in short, an enormous number, which is why angina is one of the most expensive medical problems facing our society.

We spend billions of dollars a year to deal with angina. This is not just money spent on medication and hospital costs, but money that people lose through disability. When health economists try to figure out how expensive a disease process is, they examine it from the direction not only of what it costs the health care system, but of what it costs the entire nation. They look at lost productivity (a terrible phrase, by the way), which rather coldly refers to people who can't go to work and what their absence costs the economy. They try to put a dollar figure on it, but in fact angina is probably far more expensive than that estimate, because not all loss can be measured in dollars and cents. Angina costs people the ability to enjoy their lives. That's a quantity that's hard to measure, but it is a terrible loss nonetheless.

Angina is a disease that limits your ability to exercise, and I'm using that word in the broadest sense possible. When most people hear the word *exercise* they think of playing tennis or running a marathon, but it's simpler than that. Anything the human body does that expends oxygen and causes the heart to work harder is exercise. To some people, exercise is simply walking up a flight of stairs or moving easily about the kitchen while preparing dinner. It can be something as ordinary as getting out of bed and walking to the bathroom in the morning. Most of us take these actions for granted, but people who suffer from severe angina often have great difficulty doing them. Why? Because their heart isn't getting enough oxygen to cope with the increased demand even minor exercise places upon it.

Angina is caused by plaque—hard plaque—that invades the coronary artery, making the artery more narrow and limiting the amount of blood that goes to the heart. The heart needs all the blood it can get to feed it oxygen beat after beat. When you exercise, the heart needs to work harder; it needs more oxygen. Narrowed encrusted arteries can't supply enough oxygen to the heart. Where there should be a rush of blood, there is now only a trickle; when the heart calls out for oxygen, the blood vessels can't perform their job adequately, and the heart cries out in pain.

That is the classic pain of angina.

Angina is not exactly a new disease. It has, in fact, been known almost since the dawn of recorded medical history. The symptoms of angina typically have been described as "pain that comes on with activity and is relieved by rest." The angina sufferer, however, does not usually describe the discomfort as pain, but as pressure: *"I have an elephant sitting on my chest."* If I had a dime for every time I heard that complaint in the emergency room, well, I'd probably be able to buy an elephant.

Every doctor has heard the same story. It's universal. I confess I was a doubter in medical school. But not for long. One trip to the emergency room (ER) and I was a believer. Oh, sure, an occasional angina patient complained of a boa constrictor squeezing the chest (not bad) and a few (with less imagination perhaps) simply said their chest felt "heavy," but elephants win, hands down.

Just why a pachyderm should rear its ugly trunk in the middle of this description, I don't know. But it does. Sometimes the pain radiates up to the jaw, to the teeth, or down the arm. There can be atypical pain of angina, as well. It can shoot down into the abdomen, prompting all manner of confusion. A patient will enter the emergency room and say, "Sometimes I get an upset stomach when I walk." Upon closer examination, we discover other symptoms, a history of pain or heart disease, and we understand that this is the way angina behaves in some patients. We don't really know why this happens, but it does. It's atypical angina, but it's angina nonetheless.

As with heart disease in general, angina is more common in men than in women, and in older people than younger people. It is almost always associated with disease of the coronary arteries that we can identify on an angiogram. When you inject dye into the arteries of a patient suffering from long-term chronic angina, you will usually see boulders of hard plaque sitting in the coronary arteries.

Aspirin and statins both have something to offer angina sufferers.

Statins

We know that hard plaques contain some fatty deposits as well as calcium, and that they form more often in people with high blood cholesterol level than in those whose cholesterol level is low. So we need to ask two questions: First, does lowering your blood cholesterol level prevent you from forming these rocks, and, second, if you already have them, what do the statins have to offer?

The first answer is, probably yes, and taking statins to prevent formation of hard plaque makes intuitive sense. Certainly, by lowering your cholesterol level, the statins offer the hope that you will not form these large calcified plaque deposits in your coronary arteries, and the incidence of angina should be reduced. Do we have long-term studies to prove this? Unfortunately, we're not at the point that I can say that the medical literature unequivocally shows that if you take statins for the next thirty years you will not get angina. But I think it is a reasonable assumption, and it is as reasonable as any of the diet assumptions that we have seen so far—the ones that espouse a low-cholesterol diet to aid in the prevention of angina. If anything, these diet assumptions, and the diet work that has been done over the years, are supportive evidence that statins clearly will be helpful in the prevention of angina, because, as we've already noted, diets are capable of wiggling lipid profiles by approximately 10 to 15 percent, whereas statins are profoundly more effective. If diets offer a glimmer of hope, statins offer a great deal more.

What about people who already have angina? Do the statins have something to offer? At the very least, the current literature suggests that if you lower your LDL cholesterol and triglyceride levels (another form of blood-born fat), and raise your HDL cholesterol level, you should prevent the disease from getting worse. This is, I think, the best that any diet plan with its meager cholesterol-reducing power can offer. Diets frequently claim that they're going to reduce your angina risk and make angina better. But in fact, what they are probably offering is nothing more than a slowing of the rate of progression of angina, and perhaps the potential to end it. I believe we can offer at least that much with statin therapy, and there is at least the potential to go much further—to make your angina better!

If there is any way to reduce the size of a calcium-cholesterol rock, it's going to result from dramatically lowering the level of cholesterol in your blood.

But there's more. Statins seem to have other effects as well, not directly related to plaque formation, that improve the symptoms of angina. For reasons we still don't understand completely (there's that "why" question again), statins have an impact on coronary arteries that is distinct from their cholesterol-lowering properties, and this impact makes you feel better; it reduces your symptoms. There is, therefore, at least some reason to suggest that statins, all by themselves and blood cholesterol levels notwithstanding, are simply good drugs. Indeed, the more closely we examine statins, the more interesting they become. Statins have been associated with the ability of blood vessels to change their size and grow wider in response to increased blood flow demand. They have a beneficial effect on blood clotting and on stabilizing of plaque.

In summary, here's what we can reasonably conclude about statins and angina. People with hard plaque (i.e., angina sufferers) also have soft plaque. That makes them a high-heart-attack-risk group. That means they all should be on statins to prevent heart attack stemming from what we know is its root cause: the inflammatory response associated with soft plaque. So if you are looking for a subset of people for whom our program is incredibly important, it's people with angina.

Moreover, we think that statins can stop the progression of hard plaque into your coronary arteries and thus prevent the symptoms of angina from worsening. And, for reasons we don't entirely understand, statins may help relieve the symptoms you already have. This effect happens quickly after you start taking statins, too quickly, in fact, to be explained by the notion that for some reason the statins are making your plaque smaller. The mechanism by which this happens is not entirely clear, but statins have been shown to improve the ability of blood vessels to expand and contract as needed. Since statins are a good idea for other reasons, why not take them? You might find an unexpected benefit: Your angina might be less severe.

Simply put, virtually everyone who suffers from angina (except those with some clear contraindication, such as an obvious intolerance to the drug) should be on statins, not only because statins decrease their heart attack risk but because they may get physical relief from the pain of angina. Statins may make the elephant go away. And as anyone who has angina will tell you, that's no small accomplishment.

Aspirin

Some of the same arguments that we've made in favor of statin therapy for angina victims can be made for aspirin therapy as well. Nearly everybody with angina faces a tremendously increased risk for heart attack. Angina should be a marker, a screaming siren call, for aspirin therapy. If you have angina, you should be taking an aspirin a day—unless, of course, you have some clear contraindication.

The Swedish Angina Pectoris Aspirin Trial (*Lancet*, 1992 [vol. 340, pp. 1421–25]) revealed that in two thousand people diagnosed with angina, followed over the course of four years, aspirin treatment was associated with a one-third reduction in the rate of sudden death. The authors' unsurprising conclusion: take aspirin. How much? A very small dosage, actually. As little as 75 milligrams per day. The dosage is open to debate, but what is not open to debate is that if you have angina, you should be on aspirin. Period.

Why? Aspirin inhibits the synthesis of a number of compounds that affect the ability of the blood vessel to constrict. You don't want your blood vessels to constrict if they are already too small because they contain a lot of calcium and plaque. And if you constrict blood vessels that already have an obstruction in them, you're going to have problems. Big problems.

So, aspirin provides relief not merely because it has blood-thinning and anti-inflammatory properties, but also because it blunts vasoconstriction—it prevents blood vessels from squeezing. In this way, aspirin also makes the symptoms of angina less severe. Just as with statins, you can make the case that aspirin will not only prevent you from dying, it will also make you *feel* better. Taking aspirin is definitely a win-win scenario.

Here's a fair question: How effective is our program in helping people who have mild angina symptoms from getting worse? Is our program as good as more aggressive therapy in the treatment of mild to moderate angina? In other words, if you suffer from angina, and you follow this program—the cornerstones of which are aspirin and statins—can you, for example, prevent the need for an angioplasty or a bypass? The answer unfolding in the current literature seems to be a resounding *yes*. It may just keep you out of the catheterization suite and the operating room.

So the next thing to address is long-term benefit (you won't need surgery) versus short-term benefit (you'll feel better). New studies suggest that people who have mild to moderate angina symptoms who begin aggressive lipid-lowering therapy are as effectively treated as those who have angioplasty. In fact, one paper, published in March 2002 by Dr. David T. Nash of Upstate Medical University in Syracuse, New York, asks a very important question: "Is there a need for a moratorium on angioplasty if you have stable coronary disease?" Put another way, are we performing too many angioplasties too early on too many patients without trying aggressive lipid-lowering therapy first, and should we stop doing angioplasties for a while? According to Dr. Nash, the answer is yes. And I agree with him.

He asks for a moratorium on a procedure that occurs thirteen hundred times a day, every day in the United States. That's 474,500 per year. Nearly half a million! Instead, why not try something less costly and less invasive? Why not try therapy that lowers LDL cholesterol level for a minimum of six weeks? And that's what an increasing number of physicians are suggesting: get your lipid level down, and only then, if you continue to have symptoms of angina, consider angioplasty. In short, you don't necessarily need an angioplasty to fix your coronary arteries.

Impressive stuff. But for some reason a lot of people—both in and out of the medical community—have more confidence in machinery than in chemistry. They routinely and even cavalierly say: "No, no, just go in there and ream out my coronary arteries! Then I'll worry about my cholesterol." The new research says this is backward thinking. Treat the cholesterol first, it suggests, and then see what happens.

Few people in the medical establishment suspected this outcome. The prevailing wisdom was that if we reduced your cholesterol level, we might help you live longer and avoid a heart attack, but we'd never make your angina better.

But the lipid-lowering therapy outlined in this book does indeed have the potential to make your angina better—and perhaps even give you the chance to avoid invasive therapy.

This is not to suggest that everyone with angina can be rescued by this program. The New York Heart Association divides angina into four classes:

CLASS 1   Angina only with unusually strenuous activity
CLASS 2   Angina with slightly more prolonged or slightly
    more vigorous activity than usual (walking up a flight
    of stairs, taking a brisk walk)
CLASS 3   Angina with usual daily activity

CLASS 4 Angina at rest (inability to carry on any
physical activity without pain)

As you move up the scale, obviously conditions are getting worse. It's a good idea to use aspirin or statins with any of these classes, but in terms of avoiding angioplasty or bypass surgery, we're talking about class 1 or class 2. By the time you have angina with usual daily activity—getting out of bed, going to the bathroom or kitchen—that's an indication that your disease is so far advanced that you probably don't have time to wait for the lipid-lowering effects of statins and the anti-inflammatory properties of aspirin. But if you have class 1 or class 2 angina, embracing this program greatly increases the likelihood of your avoiding an invasive procedure.

Other Techniques

It is reasonable to ask about calcium. After all, hard plaque is made up of both lipid and calcium. Isn't there some way to get at the calcium deposits in the coronary arteries at the same time we attack the lipids?

So far, the answer seems to be no.

The only folks claiming success in ridding the arteries of harmful calcium deposits are the so-called chelation therapists. They claim that by injecting into your blood chemicals that bind calcium and carry it away, they can reduce the plaque burden in your coronary arteries.

The technique has been tested extensively. It doesn't work. Still, it is being promoted vigorously, and people are trying it.

Bad idea: It is expensive, it may be dangerous, and it doesn't help. I wish it did, but it doesn't.

Smoking

We can't leave a chapter on angina without talking a bit about smoking. Scratch that: We need to talk a lot about smoking. Although we discussed why the fact that cigarette smoking made your heart attack risk worse wasn't explained by the traditional heart attack model, the risk of smoking to angina sufferers is clear and direct.

Smoking makes you feel worse and gives you angina for a very straightforward reason, and we've understood this reason for at least the last fifty years: Smoking decreases the amount of oxygen in your blood. The heart is screaming for oxygen in angina. That's what angina pain is; the heart's shouting, "I can't breathe!"

The reason it doesn't have enough oxygen is that its blood flow is already compromised by hard plaque clogging up its arteries. The heart muscle is not getting enough oxygen-carrying blood. So each oxygen molecule on each drop of blood that does reach the heart muscle is precious. The last thing in the world you want to do if you are in this state is decrease the amount of oxygen that each drop of blood can carry. But, every time you take a puff on a cigarette, you replace some of the oxygen carried by the blood with poisonous carbon monoxide.

Think about that.

Carbon monoxide: In a fire, this is the stuff that kills people. Smoke is filled with carbon monoxide. People in fires are often forced to inhale great amounts of smoke, and they quickly poison their body with carbon monoxide. Smokers, by definition, are breathing in smoke with each drag on a cigarette. The effect, filters notwithstanding, is the same as that in a fire scene.

And when you smoke, not only are you replacing the oxygen

in the blood with carbon monoxide, but the carbon monoxide binds with hemoglobin—the oxygen-carrying molecule of the blood—much more tightly than oxygen does. So it hangs around for a long time. You can't just say to yourself, "I'm going to stop smoking now, and get more oxygen to my heart in thirty seconds." It's a long, slow excretion process, and throughout that process, the amount of oxygen in your blood will be reduced.

When we discussed cigarette smoking and heart attack, we asked a simple question with a complicated answer: *Why doesn't the carbon monoxide effect of smoking cause a heart attack right away? Why don't you take a puff of a cigarette, keel over, and die?* It doesn't happen that way with heart attack, but it sure works that way with angina. You can take a puff on a cigarette and instantly find yourself shouting, "Whoa! Get this elephant off my chest."

Despite this pain, angina sufferers still smoke. That's probably the most powerful reason I know to call cigarette smoking an addictive disease, because people continue to smoke despite the powerful disincentive: angina pain. Why would you do something that hurts so much? You wouldn't, of course, unless you were hopelessly addicted, unless you were utterly compelled to do it.

The more you smoke, and the more your angina progresses, the worse it's going to hurt. This is a disease in which cigarette smoking is outrageously insane. Here it causes you excruciating pain. There is a direct cause and effect, and you feel the consequences even as the cigarette smolders between your fingers. Smoking accelerates heart attack risk, and it also accelerates angina. Therefore—I will say it once more—you cannot, you must not, smoke. And if you are smoking, you must stop. Now!

I'm not suggesting it is easy to stop smoking. I know it's hard. It is a chemical drug addiction. But millions have stopped. Millions more must stop.

The program is not designed to eliminate the risk of smoking. No statin or aspirin (or antibiotic for that matter) treatment will keep your heart safe if you continue to smoke: no discussion allowed.

Whew, I feel better getting that off my chest—not quite an elephant, but a heavy burden nonetheless.

CHAPTER EIGHT

Diet and Exercise

A caveat before we begin: Doctors Atkins, Ornish, Pritikin, and others are popular, ethical, well-intentioned physicians whose programs are designed to help you live better, feel better, and live longer. I respect their dedication. From time to time in this chapter I will refer to Dr. Atkins as a representative of a diet philosophy that recommends that you eat more protein and less carbohydrate. I'll occasionally use Dr. Ornish's name as a shorthand for a traditional low-fat-low-cholesterol dietary approach. That being said, there's a war going on. Anyone commenting on diet and heart health had better be prepared to duck.

Someone asked Groucho once, "Are you a man or a mouse?" Groucho answered, "Put some cheese down there and see what happens."

Atkins would eat the cheese. Ornish would breathe deeply and probably reject it. I'm still looking for the rest of the trap.

Diet

Lots of people think eating an appropriate diet will lower your heart attack risk. If this is true, which diet is best? Will a low-cholesterol, high-carbohydrate diet, Ornish-like diet keep you safe? Will eating more protein and fat while restricting carbohydrates, an Atkins-like plan, let you live longer? Be careful whom you ask. People get agitated about questions like these. They occasionally throw things at each other. The question you need answered is not who can shout the loudest, or sell more books, but "Do we have any evidence to support one position or another?"

I use the term *war* advisedly. Wars are often fought over principle, or articles of faith, not cold scientific evidence. People march into battle not because of what they can prove, but because of what they believe. And the wars they fight are usually undertaken to force others to believe and act as they do.

No one is holding a gun to anyone's head and forcing his opponent to eat tofu, of course. But the sniping and artillery fire between the two main warring camps in the diet and heart disease debate are quite real. One camp, the low-fat-high-carbohydrate group, says the other, the high-protein-no-carbohydrate group, is killing America. *All that protein and fat in your diet will eventually clog up your coronary arteries and cause heart attacks*, they charge. The other group says, *Phooey! You can eat fat, just don't eat bread. Our diet is just as good as yours and our advocates have more fun!*

The low-fat-high-carbohydrate folks think theirs is the only way to achieve heart health and with it true salvation. They often combine their dietary advice with other lifestyle suggestions (learning how to breathe comes to mind; so does standing on your head and learning how to think more appropriately—I'm not making this stuff up). The high-protein-low-carbohydrate advocates scoff at the monklike monasticism of the low-fat camp and eat whatever fat they wish.

Is there a right answer here? Some folks think that a good place to start looking for the answer is the medical community. "What do doctors do when they want to lose weight and improve their blood lipid levels?" It's worth remembering that doctors a half-century ago endorsed cigarettes, so you might take their lifestyle advice with a grain of salt, even today. Still, the question deserves an answer.

I've been taking a totally unscientific survey of doctors and their favorite diets during the past few years. The results are virtually unanimous. When docs want to lose weight there is little debate. Hands down, no competition, nearly every one of them chooses an Atkins-like diet. No other program is even close. What does this mean? It means that doctors are like everyone else. They don't have a clue as to which diet is better (and I mean *better* in the bigger sense of the word, lifesaving better), but they do know that the Atkins diet does seem to promote weight loss quickly and effectively, with a minimum of effort.

And there is another, subtle question that my "hallway survey" addressed. Does the diet you choose make all that big a difference to your heart health? The classic answer is yes. But the classic answer was formulated long before we had statins. In the middle of the twentieth century, diet management was all we had to control your blood cholesterol level. It seemed obvious to try to limit your cholesterol intake, to decrease the amount of cholesterol in your bloodstream. And it seemed to work to some extent; less cholesterol in your diet did seem to make your blood a little less fatty. But as we've discussed before, "a little less fatty" wasn't necessarily good enough to save your life. "A lot less fatty" was what was needed, but diet alone wasn't going to get you there.

Still, since diet control was the only weapon they had to fight high cholesterol levels in your blood, lots of doctors became passionate about the specifics of the particular diets they were recommending. "NO FAT!" became the rallying cry for most of the health care community. Of course, it soon became clear that there was a lot of money to be made by selling low-fat-low-cholesterol food. Madison Avenue was soon plastering *low fat* and *polyunsaturated* and *low cholesterol* on billboards, food labels, and TV ads all over America.

The interesting truth was, though, that no one really thought to look carefully at other dietary approaches to cholesterol control. One, the high-protein-low-carbohydrate diet, seemed so ludicrous that folks dismissed it out of hand. It was an article of faith that fat in your diet was bad, and the less fat you ate, the healthier you'd be.

It took a long time to put these two dietary approaches to the test and match them up in a scientific trial, head to head. Meanwhile, the war raged on. It's worth remembering at this point that dietary control is a good idea. Statins work nicely to reduce your cholesterol level, but diet can help, too. And in the war against death, I'll take all the help I can get.

Why did it take so long to compare the two dietary approaches?

At the risk of being provocative, I would submit that the reason the two diets were never adequately compared to each other in a controlled scientific manner had little to do with science. It came down to the fact that the people supporting each of these dietary approaches to controlling heart disease and lowering heart attack risk were (and still are) "true believers." That is to say, there seems to be no way to convince them that they may be wrong. They believe in their diet, and they believe that you should believe, too. It's not just about science; it's not that they know for a fact that their particular program is superior to another. It's about emotion and psychology and faith. History is replete with examples of such behavior. Just check out the biography of Galileo.

Some go so far as to say that if you don't follow their plan you will lose your soul! Dr. Dean Ornish once wrote an editorial in a medical journal that the fight to keep people on his program and *off statins* is nothing less than a fight for the soul of American medicine. Those were his words: "The soul of American medicine"! I don't doubt his sincerity. I just wonder about his choice of vocabulary.

The Atkins plan, on the other hand, is pretty much the "anti–Dean Ornish plan." Whereas Atkins says "Eat protein and cut carbs," Ornish says "Cut fat; eat fruits and vegetables." But the Ornish plan is more than just diet. The Ornish folks want to turn your life around. What you really ought to do, they say, is learn to control your breathing, employ stress-reduction techniques, engage in yogalike exercises. Atkins's diet plan requires less lifestyle modification, but, as with Ornish, his proponents *believe* that their diet is better, that it will help you lose weight and improve your heart attack risk profile.

Who's right? Who is telling the truth?

By now it shouldn't surprise you that truth is hard to find here.

Lots of Americans would like the Atkins plan to pan out. The Atkins book is pretty happy: *"Go on out there, eat the foods you like, and lose weight!"* That advice looks pretty good, especially if the folks from the other plan want you to live as a monk and overhaul your life.

Ornish advocates will tell you that doctors should be teaching people how to live a better life; they shouldn't be handing out pills or prescribing bacon. (A friend of mine saw a package of fried pork rinds in a store the other day. The bag screamed, "Guaranteed to contain NO carbohydrates." Did I mention that I haven't made this stuff up?)

I'm on nobody's side in this war, other than yours. I'm a pragmatist. I'm going to go with what works. If you can show me that people can maintain a monastic lifestyle, feel better, decrease their cholesterol level, lose weight, and do it easily and consistently and that everyone is going to be able to do it, then I'm with you. If you can prove to me that the Atkins diet works, and by that you mean that you'll both lose weight and improve your blood lipid profile, then the Atkins plan sounds like a good idea.

But, as all diets are, they're both likely to fail in the long term. Everybody is gung-ho when he starts a new diet, but the great majority of dieters abandon the diet within a year.

Without scientific proof that one diet is better than another, the controversy over Atkins vs. Ornish has always been more about style than about substance. They are, quite honestly, different systems of belief. You have the Gospel according to Saint Fat or the Gospel according to Saint Lean.

If you wanted to settle the issue of which diet approach is better, you might take two groups of people and give half of them one of the diets, and half of them the other diet. Then you might compare their progress and see which group did better.

First, though, you'd have to define *better*. Strangely enough, what you should want a diet to accomplish is almost exactly what you want from an exercise program. You want weight loss, you want to feel better, and you want to improve your lipid profile. You want to increase the level of your HDL cholesterol and lower the levels of your total cholesterol, LDL cholesterol, and triglycerides.

The fact that these two dietary approaches have not been compared scientifically before now is surprising. There are cynics among the medical community who believe that the studies weren't done because doing them wouldn't serve anyone's interest. As long as the answers to the important questions were unknown, then each camp could claim whatever it chose. But the head-to-head comparison research was inevitable. And it has finally been done.

In 2003, the *New England Journal of Medicine* (vol. 348, pp. 2074-81, 2082-90) published two studies comparing low-carbohydrate diets to low-fat diets in obese people, and the results were fascinating. At the end of the day, it seems, these diets are pretty much equivalent.

You may think that one sounds intrinsically healthier and "better" than the other—I'm talking, of course, about Ornish— but that's because we intuitively think that because a high cholesterol level in your blood is a bad thing, any diet high in fatty, cholesterol-containing foods has to be a bad thing. Yet that's an assumption subject to proof. From the very beginning, the Atkins camp denied that the assumption was correct, and the Ornish people argued that it was obviously correct. The Ornish diet is intuitively more logical: *Your cholesterol level is too high? Well, let's reduce the cholesterol in your diet and make the cholesterol level in your blood go down.* And it turns out you can do precisely that. But the research shows you can do the same with Atkins. Medicine is not an intuitive science (if indeed it is a "science" at all). What seems simple and obvious and correct may, in fact, turn out to be much more complicated than anyone expected it to be.

A low-fat diet doesn't necessarily keep you thin, and a high-fat diet doesn't necessarily make you fat. It's actually your totally calorie balance that matters, so you can eat lots of fat and still get thin, and you can eat lots of carbs and still get fat. As is so much of science and medicine, it's strange and wonderful and complicated.

One of the two studies in the *Journal* looked at changes in lipid level after six months in people who were on either low-fat diets or low-carbohydrate diets. The low-carbohydrate diet and low-fat diet groups fared equally well in raising HDL (good) cholesterol level and lowering overall cholesterol level. But the high-protein diet did a slightly better job of decreasing triglyceride and LDL cholesterol levels. According to this study, then, the high-protein-low-carbohydrate diet won. But the victory was by such a narrow margin, it probably isn't worth mentioning.

The second study concluded that the high-protein diet initially controlled HDL and triglyceride levels better (in other words, produced faster results), but that both diets performed about equally over the course of a year. The study concluded that the overall effect of a low-carbohydrate diet, in comparison with a low-fat diet, on the risk of coronary heart disease is "uncertain."

What does this mean to you? You should care about only one thing: whether it's possible to wiggle your heart attack risk factors enough with diet alone to keep you as safe from heart attack as possible. If the answer is yes, then your next question needs to be, Which diet approach is better? And we now realize that, according to the most pertinent and timely research, the answer is, We don't know.

That's a startling statement. After forty or fifty years of noodling and arguing about cholesterol, debating low-fat versus high-fat, we still don't know whether one diet is better than another, or whether either one provides a reasonable degree of insurance against heart attack.

After all the research, and the debate, and the noise, the one salient fact of the diet debate is this: No one knows whether diet will sufficiently affect your heart attack risk to save your life. If no one knows, the only safe assumption is that it *won't*!

We should have known this would be the result. If there were a "right" answer, we would probably have known it years ago. The kind of debate we're seeing about diets is familiar. It is "the debate that won't go away." We see debates like it all the time in the hospital. For example, you can spark one on rounds in the ICU if you ask, "Is it preferable to give intravenous sugar water, salt water, or albumin to a postoperative patient?" You can argue about this for hours on end. And doctors do. It's one of their chief hobbies. But if you actually say to them, "You know, this has been researched forever, and if there were a right answer, we'd know it and we wouldn't be having this discussion," they often stop and say, "You're right."

If we knew for certain that Atkins or Ornish is right, we wouldn't be arguing. Our argument really isn't Atkins versus Ornish at all. I can give you more data comparing the programs, but that won't answer the real question you need addressed: In this day and age, is diet alone, as a therapy, sufficient to keep you as safe from heart attack as you can be? The answer here is unequivocal, and it is clear, and in my opinion the debate on this is over:

NO!

You can argue to the point of exhaustion. You want to go on the Atkins diet? Fine, go ahead. Eat all the pork roast you'd like. Order the bacon double cheeseburger (without the bun). You want to embrace Ornish? Great. Start planting that organic lettuce and head for the yoga studio. I don't think there's a dime's worth of difference in terms of where you'll be at the end of the day. Because at the end of the day you'll probably be off the diet. That's what people do with diets. But if you want to prevent premature death due to heart attack, you can't rely exclusively on Ornish, and you shouldn't rely exclusively on Atkins. Primarily, you should rely on chemistry. You need a cholesterol hammer that is bigger, more powerful than any hammer provided by any diet. You need statins.

Are there some things you can say about diet that are good? Absolutely. Some people *feel* better on an Atkins diet. If that's the case, by all means, use it. Some people feel better on an Ornish diet. Lots of people do, in fact. We know that not only do these diets affect your lipid profile—and that does provide some benefit in terms of heart disease risk—but they also affect something else. They affect your body weight. As you will see at the end of this book, in our self-test, body weight is an independent risk factor for heart disease, and both of these diets, if you stick with them, will reduce your total body weight and body mass index. Thinner people have a lower heart attack risk. So, by all means, lose weight.

I said earlier that I am a pragmatist, and that if you held a gun to my head and ordered me to follow a particular diet, I'd probably do what most doctors do. But I don't see any objective reason to prefer one diet to another right now. My personal preference is to eat sensibly and happily and to take a statin and an aspirin. Do I think the soul of American medicine rests on taking a monastic approach to diet and exercise, or on convincing people to change who and what they are and how they want to live? No, I do not. Do I think we've lost our soul because we've found a better way to reduce heart disease risk? I do not. I think the soul of American medicine is to be found in helping people live a better life and to live it as they want. As far as I can tell, giving somebody a statin and allowing that person to live a freer life and to engage in more options is better.

Good to the Last Drop?

Since we're talking about diet and its implications, it's appropriate here to say something about coffee, long a subject of debate among cardiologists. Caffeine is a stimulant, and coffee is loaded with caffeine. Doctors often wonder, quite reasonably, whether we are doing any damage to our cardiovascular health when we drink coffee.

When I was growing up, there were people in the medical community who used to tell all their patients that coffee is bad for you. At the same time, doctors were, and remain, among the largest consumers of coffee, per capita, I've ever seen. Personally, I didn't start drinking coffee until I was an intern. (You try going to work at five in the morning and getting home at nine at night, in addition to taking "call"; see whether you can do that without coffee.) It was not unusual to see a doctor walking down the hall, carrying a steaming Styrofoam cup, lecturing a patient about the dangers of caffeine. Well, it turns out, after a lot of research, that it's probably okay to drink a moderate amount of coffee. Unless you have serious problems, for example, an arrhythmia, it's highly unlikely that a couple of cups of coffee are going to do you any harm.

So drink up.

Exercise

There is a lot less controversy about exercise, thank goodness.

The goal of any exercise program is to improve overall fitness. For our purposes, though, we're talking primarily about lowering your heart attack risk. In order to accomplish that goal, we need an exercise program that provides a few very specific effects. Clearly, as with diet, we want to lower your total body weight and improve your lipid profile.

Moreover, there is a benefit claimed by exercise advocates that needs to be examined: by increasing fitness, and increasing the efficiency of blood delivery to the tissues, they claim, the body can be "trained" not only to use oxygen better but to tolerate a lack of oxygen better. We know that heart disease and heart attack are diseases of oxygen deprivation; therefore, if we could help the body to process oxygen more efficiently, heart attack would be less likely, and angina less severe. Recovery from both would be quicker and less painful.

Does exercise live up to these claims? To a large degree, the answer is yes.

Does exercise lower your total body weight? Yes, if you eat less. You have to combine diet and exercise programs to get the complete effect, but it's fair to say that exercise is an integral part of a heart-healthy program.

Does exercise alone affect your lipid profile? Surprisingly enough, it does. What kind of exercise are we talking about? As we've long suspected, the classic aerobic exercises work best.

Researchers have studied the effects of exercise on people's lipid profiles. You can make HDL level go up anywhere from 4 to 43 percent, depending on the study you're looking at. These changes can be seen not only in people who are highly trained (serious athletes, for example), but also in people who are just reasonably fit. Endurance athletes, for example, typically have an HDL level 40 to 50 percent higher than that of people who don't exercise; their triglyceride level is roughly 20 percent lower than that of sedentary people. LDL cholesterol level is as much 10 percent lower.

The changes in serum lipid levels are impressive. In addition, exercise changes another variable that diet does not. People who exercise a lot tend to control their blood pressure better than those who don't. And we know that blood pressure is another risk factor for heart attack. Again, we don't know why exercise improves your blood pressure control. We simply know that it does. And that control is another reason why exercise is undeniably good for you.

Let's take it one step further, and ask the $64,000 question (I guess today it would be the $64 million question). Is there a way to show that exercise alone can decrease your risk of death due to heart attack? You might reason as follows: *I'm going to exercise, then I'll reduce my blood pressure and improve my lipid profile, and so I'll reduce my heart attack risk.*

Rather than extrapolate this way, I'd prefer that someone study the question and see whether people who exercise have fewer heart attacks and a lower death rate. That's a set of observable phenomena. We don't need Sherlock Holmes here, reasoning from first principles. Instead we need an investigator to design a clinical study.

Luckily, there is some good scientific evidence available, including a study that appeared in the January 2000 edition of *Medical Clinics of North America*, in which exercise contributed to a 25 percent reduction in the mortality rate among four thousand patients with demonstrated heart disease.

To me, that's impressive. It shows that exercise not only makes you feel better, but decreases your likelihood of death.

So, in sum, what are the effects of exercise? Lower blood pressure, probably fewer angina symptoms, an improved lipid profile, and a modification of body weight and composition, resulting in a preferable body mass index. Not only that, but regular exercise decreases stress and anxiety and improves the quality of your life. For all of these reasons, exercise is a good thing.

There are caveats, of course. It would be very easy for me to say, *"Everybody, I mean everybody—couch potatoes included—get up off your butt! Put on your running shoes and get out the door!"* In truth, however, a certain number of these people would keel over and die. So, although it can be demonstrated that, overall, exercise is good for you and good for your heart, there are some people for whom a sudden rigorous exercise program would prove dangerous, and perhaps even deadly. It's not as easy to say that everybody should exercise as it is to say that everybody should lose weight.

Some people, those in the high-heart-attack-risk group, for example, should talk to their doctor before going out and running ten miles. But if you and your doctor can work out an exercise program that gradually increases the amount of aerobic exercise you do, the benefits to you in the long run (well, maybe the pun was intended) will be substantial.

And remember, you don't have to run a marathon to get exercise. You simply need to get up and move. Walking is a terrific idea.

As much as I'm an advocate of exercise, it can't, on its own, replace the program outlined in this book. Why not? For the same reason that a diet program is insufficient: It won't wiggle your cholesterol level enough to make as much difference as you'd like. It won't decrease your inflammatory response enough. Is it good to do exercise in combination with following our program? Sure it is. You want to lose weight. You want all the help you can get with your lipid profile. You'd like your blood pressure to be lower. And, of course, you want your mood to be better.

But is diet enough? Is exercise enough? No.

CHAPTER NINE

The Herbal Option

*You know, the proof of something may be that myriads have
believed it, but they also believed that the world was flat.*
—MARK TWAIN

*One day when I was little, my parents were having a party.
I went around to all the adults and I said, "Drink this, it'll make you
taller. It's magic." So they all drank it, and said, "How cute, how
weird." Then I snuck off into the room where their coats were
kept, and hemmed everyone's sleeves.*
—STEVEN WRIGHT

Throughout my career as a journalist, and as a doctor—although as a journalist I've had far more power to work ill in terms of public relations—I have tried to avoid raising false hope because it's really a dangerous commodity. To that end, there were some stories I simply would not do, even if they were seemingly backed up by large university studies. If I had a dollar for every story I did not do—*We now have the handle on Alzheimer's disease! The cure is just around the corner!* Or, *We've found the obesity gene! Everyone's going to be skinny tomorrow*—I might be a very wealthy man. I'd also be a man adrift, without a moral compass.

As a journalist, you can cast a skeptical eye on health claims; it's your job. But even then, your audience all too often sees and hears only what it wants to see and hear. This is, in fact, true to some degree of herbal stories, as well. Let's say I decide to do a news story that suggests the possibility that eating crabgrass will cure heart disease. I could suffuse this story with all of the quizzical disbelief you want, but at the end of the day, people will say, "Salgo did a story on crabgrass and heart disease!" They will take from that story only what they want to take, and chances are, what they want is to believe that crabgrass will cure heart disease. After all, it's free.

For that reason, you have to be careful when you discuss herbal remedies. You don't want to ignore them, not least because some of them probably work. But it's very dangerous to wade into this morass of information, semi-information, and poorly studied information and assume that what you see and hear is true.

What is really needed here, even for those of us who would like to see more herbals found effective, is good, sound scientific inquiry. Giving something to twenty people and saying "Chew on it and tell me how you feel," then writing it all up, is not good science. There are protocols for this kind of research, and they force you to examine your results with an extraordinary degree of accuracy and objectivity. Just because you would like herbal remedies to work, it doesn't follow that they do. I would love to be able to go into my garden, pick up a rutabaga, eat it, and live forever. Unfortunately, reality usually intervenes. Reality tends to be uncomfortable. So you have to be careful when you observe something, because if you don't observe carefully, you can draw the wrong conclusion. Or, as Einstein said, "Reality is merely an illusion, albeit a very persistent one."

So I'm at the opposite end of the spectrum from the holistic folks and the "Natural remedies are best" crowd. Their approach is basically *Don't do the aspirin, don't take statins, you'll still live a better life.* It may be a better life for them. They may be very happy eating brown rice and mung bean and chanting all the time (they may even be sharpening razor blades under their pyramids), but I would like to have a more fulfilling, less restrictive life. To me, one of the benefits of twenty-first-century technology is sophisticated medicine. I know that's not the politically correct thing to say, but I'm grateful that we have pills that can make life better, that can help us live longer and avoid heart disease without sacrificing everything we enjoy. Of course you should exercise and eat a reasonable diet; I really don't think you want to start off every day with a slab of bacon and a five-egg omelette. But it has become all too fashionable to paint high-tech medicine with a broad unflattering brush: *Oh, look what the doctors and scientists are doing to the world! Isn't it awful?* In a word, no.

We've reached a point when too many people for some reason assume that all technology is evil. They scoff at statins and assume that even aspirin is bad. Well, I'm here to suggest that you keep an open mind about these things, because twenty-first-century medication is offering you a cornucopia of choices. If you use it wisely, and you pick and choose and do what you want with it, you can avail yourself of the good stuff. And there is a lot of good stuff out there that will allow you to live much longer, live much better, and enjoy your life while you're doing it. That being said, I think it's important to address the issue of herbal supplements and alternatives, because there are so-called natural products on the marketplace that can be substituted for some of the products we have discussed in this book. There are herbal products that claim to lower-cholesterol level and prevent heart disease and heart attack. There are herbals that have anti-inflammatory properties. I've been saying throughout this entire book that a great deal of modern medicine is based on herbals (aspirin and statins are, in fact, two major examples). In fact, it is the conceit of doctors in the late twentieth and early twenty-first centuries that we can make medications in the laboratory, that we understand the active ingredients, that a pill works, and we know how it works because we've analyzed it to death. When you look at the history of medicine, you find that this medical hubris is misplaced.

Throughout history medicinals have been obtained through natural sources, and many of our most trusted drugs, including the two we've discussed ad nauseam in this book, aspirins and statins, are herbals at their core, to their bones. Whether it's willow bark or it's fungi, we are talking about looking in the natural world for substances that can benefit human physiological processes. That's been the mantra (and acceptable practice) among drug companies for generations. Sea captains in the past, and airline pilots more recently, were routinely asked to take home botanical samples from wherever they traveled in the world. These samples were then grown and tested to determine whether they had any effect on disease.

Herbal medicine is hardly new, often works, and is largely uninvestigated. The bottom line on this chapter is, "There are more things on heaven and earth, Horatio, than are dreamt of in your philosophy," or, in this case, in your doctor's textbook. And you might choose to investigate some of these.

Health care is, or should be, all about choices. You can take an herbal such as Cholestin, which may indeed lower your cholesterol level, and save you a significant amount of money. Whether you want to or not is another matter altogether. There are issues of contamination and purity in these herbals that you will have to evaluate. Herbals do not go down the FDA-approval pipeline. They are not manufactured in a laboratory beaker, purified, and pristine with an eye toward FDA inspection and approval. These are substances that are available through the natural foods market. Not only that, but you are going to find herbal advocates who will tell you that the purification process involved in manufacturing FDA-approved drugs, which often narrows down the efficacious element in any one of these products to a single chemical, may be counterproductive. They'll suggest that there are lots of elements in these compounds that we don't completely understand, but that removing them from the formulation might not be a good idea. Conversely, you will find that there is a philosophy among doctors that argues that the more we know about a specific ingredient, the more we study it, the safer it is. That's in counterdistinction to the beliefs of people who say, "Nature is good, nature is wonderful, eat more nature, and you will be healthier."

It's all very confusing. Most of us are taught to believe that indeed natural is good. Madison Avenue tells us so—often right on the back of our favorite breakfast cereal. Generally speaking, natural is good, but you need to realize that not everything that's natural is safe. Sometimes natural can kill you. In fact, over many years one of the great talents of healers and shamans has been to know how to dose natural substances. Digitalis, a heart drug, was obtained from foxglove, a powerful poisonous plant. Take too much and you're dead. So a healer in Europe in the Middle Ages would give foxglove to make people feel better, and he would know precisely how much not to give. Some of the most powerful drugs we use in the operating room today—drugs like curare, a muscle relaxant—that are absolutely essential for surgery, were discovered because native tribes were using them to kill animals for food. If you look closely enough, you'll find that there have always been drugs that are simultaneously poisonous and efficacious. There is always a risk/benefit ratio (there it is again): too much of a good thing is not necessarily a better thing.

For some people, natural is a matter of cost. You don't need a prescription to get an herbal. You don't have to deal with an insurance company or HMO. Just walk into the health food store and pick up a bottle. Fast, easy, and cheap. Right? Well, maybe, maybe not. If you take a look at the active ingredients in a lot of these herbals, they tend to vary, not just from manufacturer to manufacturer, but from pill to pill. That's a scary thought. Moreover, the contaminants in these pills vary from lot to lot, and from manufacturer to manufacturer. This means you never really know for sure what you're getting in an herbal pill. Some of the contaminants that have been found in herbal medicines include microorganisms such as *Staphylococcus, Salmonella, Escherichia coli*, microbacterial toxins, even pesticides! Will you ever find this stuff in a product that has made it through the FDA approval process? Probably not. As I've said, there are aspects of the FDA approval process (part of that creaky medical bureaucracy I've talked about) that bother me, but its commitment to safety and purity is not one of them. I'm not saying this information should prevent you from walking the herbal path; I simply think that you should have information, and that you should be aware of what you're getting into. And I think you should be a bit more careful than you've probably been led to believe.

Heart-Healthy Herbals
CHOLESTIN

The first class of herbals we're going to discuss is the group that seems to affect cholesterol or has a reputation for affecting cholesterol. The big hitter here is Cholestin. Other names by which this is known are Went Yeast and Monascus Purpureus. Is Cholestin effective? Study after study has shown that it is. Tables in the medical literature in reputable journals indicate that

Cholestin is in fact every bit as efficacious as some commercial statins.

Cholestin is a natural product that, as were the first statins, is distilled from fungi. It's a fermented product. In a sense, Cholestin is the initial statin. It works, and it works well. Using it is significantly cheaper than going to your drugstore and ordering a commercial statin produced by one of the major pharmaceutical companies. The question then becomes, Is it a viable alternative to the commercial products? And the short answer is yes. But the point is actually more complicated than that.

Cholestin, a fermented product that has been used for centuries in Asia, contains starch, protein, fiber, and at least eight different statin compounds all mixed together. This is not your standard high-octane cholesterol-reducing drugstore-bought statin. Chinese studies claim the product reduced cholesterol levels by anywhere from 11 to 32 percent, and this claim has been verified by numerous American studies. In terms of efficacy, the results are similar to those obtained with commercially available drugs, and that isn't all that shocking since the active ingredients are basically the same. But remember, if you are taking Cholestin, you are, in effect, taking a statin of questionable strength and purity without a prescription. You are not being monitored by a doctor, and what doctors are watching for, as we've said, are the known side effects of statins: liver, kidney, and muscle problems.

That's my caveat. So, are you running a substantial risk by taking Cholestin as a health food or a nutriceutical, as opposed to one of the commercially prepared statins? Probably not. If that's the way you want to go, I have very little reason to object to it. That said, if you are like me, a type A personality, somebody who would like to know exactly how much he's taking and how the pill is prepared and to be convinced that within this pill there are no adulterants or toxins, other than that which I know about from the FDA and drug company labs, then you should use one of the commercially prepared statins.

Cholestin will save you some money, and it will save you the potential aggravation of negotiating with a health care system that might not think you need any help with your cholesterol level. I've already recommended that statins be made available over the counter in dosages similar to that of Cholestin, so that gives me a very thin reed upon which to base any recommendation against Cholestin and in favor of a drug company product. The purity issue is real, the variability issue, pill to pill, is real. But Cholestin works. There is no question about that.

GARLIC

Extract of garlic, *Allium sativum*, is also known as "poor man's treacle" (*treacle* is defined by *Webster's* as "a medicinal compound formerly used as an antidote for poison"; the poison, in this case, is heart disease). You may have heard an awful lot about garlic extract in radio and television commercials. It's being pitched vigorously by celebrities who claim to use it to prevent heart disease. But the unfortunate truth is that most studies indicate that garlic is simply not very effective as a lipid-lowering agent. You can get garlic as an oil or in pill form. It's safe, and there are no documented drug interaction problems. Unfortunately, it's just not going to do much, if anything, to lower your cholesterol level. If you want to put it on your food, go right ahead. I think it tastes great. But if you're looking for something that will decrease your risk of heart attack by reducing the amount of lipid in your blood, garlic isn't it.

SOY PROTEIN

Soy protein, the foundation of many vegetarian diets, does seem to have some cholesterol level–reducing effect. Studies have shown that a diet rich in soy protein can reduce total cholesterol level by as much as 5 to 9 percent. And it may even decrease LDL cholesterol level by 13 percent. Why? Apparently, in some people, soy protein has the ability to change the way the liver metabolizes cholesterol. The extent to which this change occurs varies widely, but there is no denying that soy has some efficacy. Soy may also decrease cholesterol absorption—either in the stomach or in the gut. There is also something else at work here. People usually eat soy as a meat substitute. Soy protein, if substituted for animal fat, lowers your total cholesterol level. So we're not dealing with an entirely pure effect here. Part of the reason it works is almost certainly that it's replacing other fat in your diet, and that muddies the scientific water just a bit. Nevertheless, there is sufficient evidence to suggest that there is an added effect of soy protein, over and above the fat-substitution effect, that helps lower your cholesterol level. And that effect is sufficient to consider soy protein as an herbal or nutritional weapon against heart disease.

How much soy protein is required to achieve significant results? Quite a bit, actually. The average daily dosage is 25 grams. One cup of soy milk, for example, contains anywhere from 3 to 10 grams of soy protein. Four ounces of tofu contains 5 to 13 grams; a half-cup of textured soy protein, 6 to 11 grams; a half-cup of soy flour, 20 grams. So you need a lot. But it works— at least a little bit. It also seems to be tolerated reasonably well. Some people have minor side effects when they suddenly increase the amount of soy protein in their diet—diarrhea and stomach pain are the most common complaints—but there are no major issues involving drug interaction.

GUGULIPID

Also known as guggalgum or commiphora momol and widely used in India, gugulipid is an herbal designed to treat high cholesterol level. At least two controlled studies, published in India but not replicated in the West, have shown gugulipid reduces cholesterol level by as much as 22 percent. That is an extremely impressive number; however, the only evidence was gleaned from small and very limited studies, so it's hard to say with any degree of certainty whether the product truly works. Side effects appear to be minimal and the cost for a 75-milligram dose is roughly half of the cost of statins. On the surface, at least, gugulipid seems to be a promising nutraceutical, but it is not yet widely available, and there are variability issues. Bottom line: too early to tell for sure.

UBIQUINONE

Also known as *Coenzyme Q10*, ubiquinone is not a cholesterol-lowering agent but rather an herbal, taken in liquid or capsule form, that is marketed as a heart-healthy nutriceutical. This use of this drug (and it is a drug, regardless of its herbal base) is fairly widespread, and that concerns me a bit, because, theoretically at least, Q10 can be dangerous. This is a drug used by people with heart failure, ostensibly to make them "feel" better. And it probably does make them feel better. When you have heart failure, fluid begins to accumulate in your heart and lungs and legs. This makes you feel sick and short of breath. Q10 seems to make the heart beat more efficiently and makes it fail less, thus making your lungs drier, so you can breathe more easily; it probably helps the edema in your legs go away, too.

Q10 is also a diuretic, insofar as that if your heart pumps harder, and you get more fluid to your kidneys, you excrete that fluid. That's all good, and in fact there is at least one other drug that is herbal-based that does essentially the same sort of thing: digitalis. One of the problems with Q10 is that there have been no long-term studies on how it affects life span; however, such studies have been performed on digitalis. Digitalis has been used for centuries and is presumed to be heart-healthy. It makes you feel better, but it doesn't increase your life span. The reason for that, we think, is that you don't get something for nothing. If you make your heart work harder, that is to say, fail less, you have to increase its oxygen consumption. That can be a problem.

The reason many people have heart failure is that there is not enough oxygen feeding the heart to begin with. They have serious vascular disease, heart disease, which limits the amount of oxygen-carrying blood that reaches the heart. If you're trying to provoke the heart to beat harder, without enough fuel, eventually you're going to have trouble, and that could lead to more damage over time, or, even worse, a heart attack. I'm not saying Q10 has been proven to do this, but many doctors who have been looking at digitalis research worry a little about the risks of giving Q10 to heart failure patients.

HAWTHORN

Hawthorn, available as a dry extract or liquid, is a very interesting drug, primarily because it looks as though it may have ACE-inhibitor-like effects. ACE inhibitors are antihypertensive drugs that dilate the blood vessels. This is a good thing for someone with heart disease. Preliminary indications are that hawthorn may be a pretty good example of a heart-healthy nutriceutical, although we don't know for sure. It's been approved for use in Germany, and doctors in Asia have long prescribed it for mild cases of congestive heart failure.

How does hawthorn help the heart? Rather than prodding the

heart into working harder, it dilates the blood vessels into which the heart is beating; this dilatation of the vessels allows the heart to pump the same amount of blood while working *less* hard.

Again, it's a bit early to tell, but hawthorn is an herbal product that seems to be promising.

OMEGA-3 OILS

Fish oils rich in polyunsaturated fats have been found to lower plasma triglyceride levels and have anticlotting properties (and perhaps even anti-inflammatory properties). We know through anecdotes at the very least that cultures whose diet is rich in these fish oils (Mediterranean cultures, Aleut populations, the Japanese before they started eating too much beef) have lower heart disease rates. Now, is that because of the oils themselves? Are they active in some way? Or is it because the fish oil is replacing other (bad) oils in their diet? As with soy protein, the answer is, Probably some combination of the two. But the oils are active and they probably do have some role in making your heart healthy and lowering your cholesterol level. It's reasonable to eat a diet that is high in these fish oils.

Salmon is a good place to find these so-called essential oils (they're essential oils because the human body is incapable of generating them on its own). Recommended dosages for people who believe in the merits of omega-3 oils are anywhere from 1,800 to 15,000 milligrams a day. That's a broad range. At the upper end, it's also a pretty steep figure, one that most people will find nearly impossible to reach without supplements. Typically, whenever I see this kind of wide variation in dosage, I know that scientists are still knee-deep in research, so I would not recommend that you go out and gobble 15,000 milligrams of omega-3 oil each day. If you think you're not getting enough of it in your diet, you should err on the low side, simply because we don't really know what's going on yet. Personally, I don't take omega-3 supplements, but I do believe a diet high in seafood, and high in these essential oils, is a good idea.

Anti-inflammatories

We have discussed at length the inflammatory response, and why it is so important to understanding the new model of heart disease. So we should also look at some of the herbal anti-inflammatory products on the market. There is, however, just one problem. We already have the granddaddy of them all, and it's available right now, over the counter. I'm referring, of course, to aspirin.

No doubt you will be able to find willow bark or willow extract in health food stores, and either of those probably works because we know that the salicylates in aspirin are derived from the same chemicals found in willow. Nevertheless, if I were asked to choose between chewing willow bark or taking an aspirin a day, I'd opt for aspirin. On this point, I feel pretty strongly that I'd be making the right decision. Aspirin is so cheap and effective that I personally see no reason to turn to willow bark to get my dosage of aspirin.

Aspirin was chemically derived from something that was originally an herbal remedy for pain and fever—the bark of the willow plant. Aspirin works. Why go further? You have to find something that works better than aspirin and has fewer side effects to interest me in using it instead of aspirin. Aspirin is the gold standard, and for an herbal anti-inflammatory to meet that standard, it has to be tested against aspirin. The first thing I can tell you is that almost nothing has been tested in this manner. Almost all of these anti-inflammatory herbals have been studied against placebos, sugar pills, or studied in terms of subjective response without any good hard objective control.

Herbal anti-inflammatory products, in my opinion, face a Sisyphean task. They have to beat aspirin. We know aspirin works; we know it has hundreds of years of experience and research to recommend it. It meets all the criteria that I like in a drug: it's been studied, it's been proved effective, it addresses a mechanism that is probably the root cause of the heart attack problem, it's cheap, and it's available everywhere. You'll have to go a long way to convince me that the herbal anti-inflammatories out there are better simply because they travel directly from the farm to you, still shaking the dirt off their roots. That doesn't cut it for me. Anyone who believes these products are better than aspirin should be eager to prove that. If that can be done, I will be eager to believe it. To date, that hasn't happened.

So why not drop the subject? Again, it's about choice. It's about having access to information and using it as you see fit. Since some of these products have become relatively commonplace, they're worth mentioning in this space. Too, there is the issue of sensitivity. Some people do not tolerate aspirin well, and for these people, perhaps an herbal anti-inflammatory product makes sense. Certainly there is some scientific evidence that some of these products have active ingredients, so if you have documented sensitivity to aspirin, you can try these. Do they work? We don't really know and probably won't know for quite some time, but it's reasonable to ask, since this inflammatory model for heart disease is so new, whether any of the herbals have been tested in terms of anti-inflammatory activity and what their effect on heart disease is. At the present time, the answer is no; that isn't all that surprising when you consider that aspirin itself has only been studied in this context recently.

The first consideration with all of the herbal anti-inflammatories is to see whether they really are anti-inflammatory agents. Most of them have been tested against the obvious diseases that are known to have an inflammatory component, such as arthritis and autoimmune diseases. If they seem to be anti-inflammatory in nature and they are effective against arthritis, lupus, and other autoimmune diseases, it may be reasonable to try them to fight the inflammatory component in heart disease. Is there reason to think that they may offer something in addition to what aspirin offers, some secret, as yet undiscovered benefit? The answer is complicated. These herbals are complex compounds, and since to this day we don't know all of the effects of aspirin, despite the fact that it's been very well studied, there may indeed be additional properties of these other anti-inflammatories that make them better than, or at least different from, aspirin. The truth is, we just don't know.

With that in mind, here are a few of the better-known herbal products that purport to have anti-inflammatory properties, with a comment on each.

EVENING PRIMROSE OIL

Tested against placebo in studies to determine whether duration of pain and morning stiffness were decreased: no marked discernible difference found.

BLACK CURRANT SEED OIL

Tested against placebo to determine changes in morning stiffness, reduction in pain, and increase of grip strength: some efficacy found.

BORAGE SEED OIL

Tested against placebo to measure changes in morning stiffness, activity level, and reduction in pain: some significant improvements found, specifically in response to health assessment questionnaires focusing on joint tenderness.

HARPAGOPHYTUM EXTRACT

Tested for short periods against placebo: some significant improvements found.

WILLOW BARK EXTRACT

An aspirinlike compound tested against placebo: no great surprise—it works.

PHYTODOLOR

Tested against placebo: some improvement in symptoms found.

GAMMALINOLEIC ACID

A known anti-inflammatory, found in both borage seed oil and black currant seed oil: some efficacy noted.

TRIPTERYGIUM WILFORDII HOOK F (TWHF)

An Asian anti-inflammatory, immunosuppressive drug, TwHF is a vinelike plant that grows wild in China. It seems to have some effective properties, although you should know that the major use of this agent in China, outside traditional medicine, is as an insecticide. Again, this points out the need to educate yourself and to be aware that natural does not always mean better or safer.

Research indicates that TwHF is indeed an interesting drug, but research also notes that this is not a drug to be taking without medical supervision; it has to be monitored to prevent severe intoxication. In specific, for patients with diminished function of the kidneys, long-term treatment may result in damage to the reproductive system. That's not a drug I would want to be on.

VITAMIN E

Readily available over the counter, vitamin E has become one of the most popular herbal products. You've probably heard a lot of wonderful claims about vitamin E—that it's an antioxidant—that is, a free-radical scavenger; that it protects lipids in the heart; and that it decreases the rate of heart disease (a lot of this sounds vague to me, too). Well, the jury is still out on all of that. Do some homework and you'll find papers that claim vitamin E is astoundingly and broadly effective, and these are serious studies. You'll also find papers that state, unequivocally, that vitamin E simply doesn't work. What do I know? I know for sure that it works on skin conditions, but if you take it for heart disease, to prevent heart attack, you may be wasting your money.

The thinking is that somehow the oxidation of lipids in the body leads them to be more harmful than they would otherwise be, and vitamin E supposedly protects lipids from oxidation and in so doing may help prevent the formation of arterial plaque. That's the theory. A good characteristic of vitamin E is that it can be purchased from reputable suppliers with less concern for toxicity than for many other herbal products. Whether it prevents heart disease or cancer, whether it really accomplishes any of the things its supporters claim that it does, we don't know for sure. The best I can say is that it's unproved. The worst I can say is that if you take too much of anything, it can be potentially dangerous (some studies note warnings about interactions between vitamin E and other drugs, including Coumadin), and it certainly is dangerous to your pocketbook.

The bottom line on herbals is that some of them work. Surprisingly enough, you'll find that doctors are willing to recommend a lot of this stuff. But a disturbing percentage of herbal products are unproven, untested, and harmful. They contain adulterants and ingredients that are not listed on the label. So do your homework and talk to your doctor.

CHAPTER TEN

Testing

I was driving home from the hospital one evening not long ago, listening to a sports talk show on a very popular mainstream radio station. They were about to break for a commercial, and I was about to switch away and check out the rest of the dial, when I was shocked to hear a one-minute ad for an absurd testing program. I can't remember the exact wording, but the thrust of the promotion was this: *"Get a CT scan of your body! Or an MRI! And if you get an abdominal scan, for a limited time only, we'll throw in a heart scan—FREE!"* All that was missing was a plug for the "Chop-O-Matic," or "Ginsu, the miracle knife."

Why would an otherwise healthy man or woman respond to such a bizarre advertising campaign? Because we, the doctors of America, told them to—not directly, of course, but by implication. We have been so technology-driven, and so technology-blinded, that we have trumpeted the value of the latest high-tech test as the best way to prevent death and destruction. If the sixties were marked by the slogan "Better Living Through

Chemistry" (if you don't remember it, or weren't alive at the time, don't worry; it didn't make much sense then either; that's probably why the slogan was adopted by the counterculture), then the first years of the twenty-first century might be characterized by "Better Living Through Medical Technology."

We all fear the unknown. Our new testing machines, then, must be a way to see into the darkness, and shine a light into the areas where danger may be lurking in the human body. Maybe there's a small spot on your lung, a tiny blockage in your coronary artery, a microscopic blood vessel waiting to pop in your brain. And if you catch it early with magnetic resonance imaging (MRI), or a computed tomography (CT) scan, or a stress test, you can save your life. Something evil may be lurking in there, and we have to find it. Now! The problem is, these tests are terrifically expensive, and not all that terrific at finding significant disease before it causes trouble. And then, there are the disturbing statistics to consider. The vast majority of these studies will turn up absolutely nothing, while costing an arm and a leg. Used indiscriminately they can bankrupt our nation's health care budget while saving very few lives.

But the other side of the argument is seductive. "Don't care about statistics, or national health care budgets," the small voice in our head whispers. "This test may save *your* life right now. You've got the money. Go for it."

That's why this stuff is marketed day and night, and why it's finding customers.

Some corporations have been offering what is known as "executive screening" for years. "Executive screening" is a set of medical tests—some invasive, some not so invasive—offered to upper-echelon employees as an executive "perk." Executive screening is an extremely expensive program, because you're basically buckshotting tests at people without symptoms who shouldn't have anything wrong with them (except maybe a severe case of hyperinflated wallet syndrome). It's called executive screening because they are, after all, the only people the corporate boards think are worth the expense. It's a costly benefit, and it is rarely offered to blue-collar workers.

But the ironic truth is, the blue-collar workers are getting the better deal. They are not subjecting themselves to tests they don't need. They are not going to pay for them, either out of their pockets directly or out of their expensive compensation packages, and they're not going to suffer the side effects of the tests either.

The executive screening concept is a bad deal for the average American, and it's a bad deal for the executive elite. In fact, it's not suitable for anyone. Still, it's being marketed, and people are buying it.

There is another, more subtle cost to "well-adult screening," and it's difficult to quantify. Every test has a certain amount of inaccuracy associated with it. Sometimes the test will tell you that you are healthy when you are not. Sometimes it will indicate you've got trouble when you're really perfectly fine.

Both results are dangerous. And both are a terrible waste—and in this case the waste can be measured in lives lost. In the first case, when a test gives you a clean bill of health you don't deserve, you do not take actions you need to take. You assume you are healthy when you are really sick, then become sicker, and possibly die as a result. But the second result, when the test says you're less healthy than you really are, can kill you, too. A so-called false-positive finding can lead you to get other unnecessary, more invasive, and dangerous tests with side effects that can be lethal.

Waste of this magnitude has contributed dramatically to our spiraling health care costs. I can't tell you the exact percentage of the American health care budget that has gone into unnecessary well-person testing and its inevitable aftermath. No one can. But left unchecked, it will break the bank.

As you wander the hospital corridors of America and listen to the doctors who work there, you can feel the mood. There is a sense that everybody needs to be tested at all times, for everything; indeed, if we get sick, there is a tendency to lay the blame not on some quirk of fate or behavioral misstep, but rather on shoddy diagnostic work. The test didn't work, it wasn't sensitive enough, the right one wasn't ordered, or we didn't get tested in time.

How have we arrived at this point? The answer is complicated. One part of the answer that most doctors will give you immediately is "It's the fault of the damn lawyers!"

Consider the fact that doctors commonly refer to certain diagnostic procedures as "CYA tests," as in "cover your ass." I'm not joking. This is precisely the way these tests are routinely described in clinical settings. They are tests that doctors order in the hospital or office primarily because they think that if they don't order them and something goes terribly wrong with the patient, they're going to look bad in court.

The important point to understand about many of these tests, whatever they may be, is that the doctor realizes the patient doesn't need them and may even tell the patient that he or she doesn't need them. At the same time, the doctor's lawyer, implied or actual, is whispering in the doctor's ear, day and night, *"Get the test, get the test, get the test."*

This unfortunate practice has grown exponentially in the last twenty years, to the point that technology has created in the United States, and in much of the developed world, a voracious appetite for testing among doctors. Is that good or bad? Simple. It's bad. Because we are testing without clear and precise goals.

The measure of any test should be its usefulness: *What are you going to do with the result?* One of the questions you must ask yourself before you order a test is "How will I use the information the test will give me?" If the answer is "The result will be nice to know, but it's not going to change anything that I do," then what's the point of having the test?

A test must have focus; it must impart information that you can use in some meaningful way. A test should have the potential to alter the way you live, or at least the way you will combat some type of illness.

I'd like to share a dirty little secret with you. CYA tests have become so pervasive that many doctors have stopped checking the results of the tests they've ordered! That's right. The results of many of these tests, the kind ordered so casually and smoothly each Thursday night on *ER*, often are not examined. The practice has become so standard and accepted, and so costly, that it's finally being addressed. In many hospitals, medical students are now being explicitly directed to find out the results of the tests they've ordered. We, as teachers, have to drill it into medical students and residents: "If you order a test, you're responsible for knowing the result." I never thought, a generation ago when I was beginning my practice, that I'd be standing on rounds in the twenty-first century waiting for recalcitrant medical students and interns and residents to call the labs and get results of tests they forgot they had ordered! Now, I ask you, why would a doctor order a test whose results seem to be so unimportant that he wouldn't even bother to find out what they are? The answer: because it's a CYA test and its results are useless.

Are there some tests that you, as a concerned person, might want to take to find out whether you are "heart-healthy"? Yes, there are. Who should take them, what do the results mean, and what are you going to do about the results? The best way to decide is to look at each of the tests in detail.

But before we begin, I think it's reasonable to say that even without the information from *any* of the tests we are about to examine, it makes sense to begin the program in this book. The results of these tests may be nice to know, inasmuch as they may raise your alarm level about a particular problem, thus making it more likely that you will do something to fix it. But, in point of fact, you can ask a very simple question: Will a negative result of any of these tests absolve you of the need to be concerned about your heart?

The answer is no. So, with that caveat—that is, even if you get a clean bill of health on everything we're about to describe, including cholesterol profile and stress test—you still should consider taking an aspirin a day, taking a course of antibiotics, and taking a statin. Because we know that even people in the low-risk group reduce their risk of heart attack by embracing this program.

That's an important caveat, because we've already discussed that all tests involve risk. As you read forward you should constantly be assessing the risk of a particular test to you.

When assessing the merits of a particular test, the rules of logic should apply to both laypeople and physicians. *How much risk does the test involve, and is the benefit of having the test potentially going to exceed the risk of having it?* In other words, why get a test if the risk of that test is greater than the risk of the disease for which you are testing? A test has to have a favorable risk/benefit ratio, and you have to know what you're going to do with the results. And don't lose sight of the fact that a test may not give you a straightforward answer. You should think about what a "maybe" answer on a test will lead you to do as you assess its potential for harm.

Think about it: If the test result is "slightly" positive, what are you going to do next? It is possible to start testing and then find yourself following a path that will lead you to an operating room, simply because at each step of the way, the test finding was marginally positive. So you ask yourself, Do I want to go there? It's another way of saying "What the hell am I going to do with this information?"

As you get away from the easy screening tests and move toward the more invasive tests, each one ordered because the one preceding it had a "marginally positive" result, you're involving yourself in riskier and riskier medicine, not to mention increased cost. You have to examine with some care what the test will give you, what the test will not tell you, and whether or not it will impact how you behave and what the risk of your subsequent behavior will be.

With that being said, let's take a look at some of the most commonly administered cardiac tests (or those with a significant cardiac component), and weigh their relative risks and attributes.

The Annual Physical

Believe it or not, the good old standby, the annual checkup, which most people don't even consider to be a "test" in the traditional sense of the word, is probably not a great idea. It may not be a terrible idea, either, but it may be a waste of time. As you get older, a periodic visit to your doctor's office makes more sense, and there are specific times you should want to visit the doctor. But a generic visit to your doctor, for nonspecific reasons—*I was walking down the street today and was thinking, "Hey, it's time for my annual checkup,"* or your insurance will pay for it—actually does you very little good. The "pickup" on the annual exam—the discovery of something truly valuable (i.e., life-threatening)—is so small, especially in young people (younger than age forty), as to make it virtually useless.

There are reasons to go to the doctor for a so-called routine checkup, but usually these are tied to milestones that indicate that a checkup is necessary. Age is a milestone, for example. So are routine Pap smears or breast examinations, mammograms, and colonoscopy, to name a few others. Similarly, if you want to see your doctor to determine your baseline heart health at a young age, that, too, makes sense. But be clear as to why you're going to the doctor. Make sure you have a deeper reason than a desire to walk out of the office afterward and say, "I saw my doctor and got a clean bill of health, and that's all I need to do until next year."

Lipid Profile

At some point, let's say before the age of twenty-five, a doctor visit does make sense, even if you're feeling fine. And there are some tests that make sense for your doctor to order, and for you to request at that visit.

The first of these tests is for total serum cholesterol level, or a fractionated blood lipid profile, to be precise. Everyone should have one of these, preferably earlier rather than later. You are looking for four numbers: measurements of total serum cholesterol level, high-density lipoprotein level, low-density lipoprotein level, and triglyceride level. Ideally, your HDL level should be high, and your LDL and triglyceride levels should be low. The reason you want to know these numbers is that there are people who, even at a very early age, carry in their blood dangerous levels of these lipids. The higher the numbers for total serum cholesterol, LDL, and triglyceride levels, and the lower the numbers for HDL level, the more likely you are to have significant heart disease at an earlier age. Your appearance and behavioral patterns do not necessarily determine where your profile will fall. We've talked about Jim Fixx, but there are also children, teenagers, and people in their early twenties who have nasty blood lipid profiles. You'd never know it by looking at them. As a result, it's reasonable to check your lipid profile. If you find that it's askew, it should alarm you and cause you to go on our program even earlier than you might have.

The more heart disease in your family history, the earlier you should think about getting tested. If you have a strong family history of angina and heart attack, then you really have an obligation to know your lipid profile as early as possible. How early? I recommend you be checked before you turn twenty. On the other hand, if everyone in your family has lived to be ninety or one hundred years old, you can probably delay the test for ten years.

It makes sense to talk about these four tests—total cholesterol level, HDL level, LDL level, and triglyceride level—as the foundation of a heart-healthy program. Getting these tests done is completely justified. They're relatively inexpensive, they're easy to administer, and they are not dangerous or invasive. Four numbers, one little needle stick. The risk to you, the patient, is virtually zero, and the benefit could be astronomical. So I like this test—a lot.

Blood Sugar

Again, blood sugar level is a good thing to check. You should have this done when you're having your cholesterol level checked, and not merely because the results can be derived from the same needle stick. We know that diabetes affects your heart disease profile adversely. If you are predisposed to elevated blood sugar level, you have to know about it early, and you have to treat it early, not only because diabetes itself is a lethal disease, but also because it carries with it the problem of accelerated heart disease risk.

If there's one thing we know for certain about this program, it's that diabetics benefit most from aggressive lipid level lowering with statins. You have a lot to gain from knowing your blood sugar level and a lot to lose if it's too high and you don't know it. So get your blood sugar level checked. If it's abnormal, it has to be rechecked, and if it's still abnormal, not only do you need to have your diabetes treated, but you must go on the program earlier than you thought you would.

Bottom line: a low-risk test with extraordinary potential benefits.

C-Reactive Protein Test

The C-reactive protein test is controversial, and its benefits are debatable. It's extremely expensive at the moment, primarily because not many people are getting it and not many places are offering it. For many years it's been used as a research tool: Scientists and physicians have been monitoring the presence of noninflammation of the C-reactive protein, following patients over time, seeing what C-reactive protein does as patients have heart attacks, and seeing what it does afterward. It's an extraordinarily useful research tool, and one that has led us to the conclusion that in fact inflammation plays a critical part in the heart attack mystery. So the obvious question is, Why not flip it over? If C-reactive protein tells us that inflammation is the cause of heart disease, can we say that if we monitor C-reactive protein and do a routine screening test using C-reactive protein, we can spot those people at risk for high amounts of inflammation in their coronary arteries, and thus at high risk for heart attack? Or put more simply, is the C-reactive protein test ready for prime time as a mass-screening tool for heart attack risk?

You will not yet find it as an official recommendation of any medical organization, but a significant and respected group of doctors, growing by the day, say that we should be measuring C-reactive protein the same way we measure cholesterol level. Some research says it's a better indicator than serum cholesterol level for predicting heart attack risk.

That said, I can't deny that there are problems with the test. For one, because C-reactive protein measures inflammation, and there are diseases (the common cold is one) other than heart disease that produce inflammation, a random C-reactive protein evaluation is not the most specific test for heart attack risk I have ever seen.

If you have the sniffles, get a C-reactive protein test, and are told that the level is abnormally elevated, you shouldn't necessarily become alarmed and go on to have a series of tests that are progressively more dangerous. So, as a caveat, if you're going to have a C-reactive protein test, you need to be sure that you are otherwise healthy: no cold, no flu, no bronchitis—no infection, period.

But, you may ask, What about chlamydia pneumonia? If I had a chlamydia pneumonia infection, wouldn't that elevate my C-reactive protein level, and wouldn't I like to know that? The truth is, no one is really sure what C-reactive protein tells us about an acute *Chlamydia* infection. Certainly, if you have bacterial infection of your lungs, pneumonia, your C-reactive protein level will be high, but that may not be telling you anything about which bacteria are giving you trouble. And it may not be telling you anything useful about your heart health.

Still, if your C-reactive protein level is elevated, and you're not otherwise infected or suffering from one of myriad diseases that produce inflammation, then that high C-reactive protein level probably has predictive value. It is telling you that you are at increased risk for heart attack. That is what the proponents of C-reactive protein level testing argue, and they make a very compelling case for it.

On the basis of that information, I think it's reasonable to get a C-reactive protein level test, probably at the same time that your cholesterol and blood sugar levels are checked. But you need to remember the test is nonspecific and its predictive value has not been fully worked out just yet.

Genetic Studies

There are more and more studies that seem to show there are specific human genes that increase your heart attack risk. Does this mean that everyone should have genetic testing? After all, if knowledge is power, then the more you know about your genetic makeup, the better prepared you'll be to wage war on the ravages of age and illness.

Or maybe not.

Most of these genetic tests reveal nothing more concrete than a predisposition—at best, they can tell you that you are likely to be at increased risk for heart attack, not that you are definitely going to get sick and die early in life. Insofar as that prompts you to begin the program, fine, but I'm recommending that you start the program anyway. In the meantime, many genetic tests, including the one used to determine heart disease risk, are not ready to be used as screening devices. They are expensive and not widely available.

Besides, you've already got the best genetic test in the world, your family history: talk to your parents. You can't pick them, but you can talk to them. It would be worthwhile to know whether Aunt Ethyl and/or Uncle Seymour died of a heart attack before age forty. That information is vastly cheaper than genetic testing. Why do you need a zillion-dollar machine and a National Institutes of Health (NIH) grant to tell you that your entire family dropped dead of heart disease before their fiftieth birthday? If they did, do you think it might be something in your family's genes and that you, too, are at high risk for heart attack? Well, yeah.

Don't get me wrong. I'm not denying that examining the human genome is a worthwhile endeavor. But not on my dime, or my blood, right now. I can just talk to my folks.

Stress Test

The stress test is one of the staples of "executive testing," and indeed one of the most commonly employed tools of the cardiac trade. In theory it's simple and sound: get on a treadmill, crank up the speed or the incline, make your heart work harder, monitor the heart with an electrocardiogram or some other technique, and see what happens. Give everybody a stress test, proponents argue, and we'll unmask hidden heart disease in time to fix it before it kills you. Well, maybe it will, and then again, maybe it won't. No one denies the value of stress testing people with symptoms of cardiac trouble.

But there is a real problem with stress tests in asymptomatic people, and that's who we're talking about when we talk about using stress testing as a screening tool. We're asking whether people with no symptoms of heart disease, no reason to worry, should get a provocative test—and that's what this is—to try to find evidence that their heart might be in trouble by stressing it. That's why it's called a *stress test*.

Plenty of evidence indicates this strategy can lead to trouble. Let's say you get a stress test, and maybe the result shows a little abnormality, not necessarily anything to worry about, but something a little off. The next thing you know, you're getting an angiogram, and then the angiogram shows equivocal results, and you get an angioplasty, or you go to the operating room, where—look out—you get your chest cracked open. This is a classical scenario of the consequences of unnecessary testing. It happens.

Think about it. You start out with an equivocal stress test result, which leads to an equivocal result on cardiac catheterization (a dangerous test in its own right), and then nobody quite knows what to do. A lot of people—patients and physicians— simply opt for the final step of the process: *Go ahead and operate*. They just want to get it over with. Some of them die.

No coronary artery blockage is good, but the risk/benefit ratios favor treating only significant obstruction to flow. So what do you do to prevent getting into trouble? You get a stress test only when you need one. There are standards for stress testing set by the American College of Physicians, the American College of Cardiologists, and the American Heart Association. The standards divide folks into two groups. There are those people with definite indications for testing, the class I group. And then there are those for whom testing has less obvious benefit, the class II group.

Class I indications for a stress test include the following: reporting odd symptoms that may be related to heart disease, but nobody is sure; taking a look at patients with known heart disease in order to see just how functional they are, and what their prognosis is in the future; assessing how much the heart has been damaged after a heart attack; determining whether a patient is seriously impaired after surgery or angioplasty.

As you can see, three of the class I indications involve patients with known heart disease; the fourth involves a suspicion of heart disease. Clearly, the testing is not intended to be random and indiscriminate. The overriding sense of the hard-and-fast class I indications for stress testing is that virtually everybody who gets a stress test should either have heart disease or be at high suspicion for heart disease.

Then there are class II indications, and here there is a divergence of opinion. We use stress testing for people who have specific occupations, such as air traffic controllers or police officers. We use it for men and women who have specific risk factors, or we use it for guys over forty who have been couch potatoes for a while, have a little excess baggage around the middle, and suddenly want to start exercising. We observe these people under careful conditions to see, quite literally, whether they are likely to drop dead. Better to have them suffer a heart attack in the hospital than in the cockpit; at the radar screen, fire site, or crime scene; or during pickup basketball in the park.

But tell me. Do you see anywhere on this list of indications *a history of a three-piece suit, a two-martini lunch, and a house in the country as well as a penthouse in the city?* I don't see it, and I've looked at this list very carefully. I don't see "I want to know because I want to know, and I'm entitled to my executive screening." Now, if you have the money to plunk down, be my guest, but I think you're throwing that money away.

The stress test is a rather blunt instrument, and a significant number of people who don't have heart disease test positive. Then what do you do? It just bogs down the system, causing unnecessary worry and concern and a lot of unnecessary further testing. Oh, and by the way, approximately one of every ten thousand people who have a stress test drops dead.

Something to keep in mind.

Electrocardiogram

An old standby, the electrocardiogram does have some predictive value, but not much. It's a pretty poor crystal ball. A cardiogram tells you where you are "now." It can show you whether or not you're having a heart attack at any given moment. It can suggest you've had a heart attack sometime in the past. But it's much more difficult—in fact, it's a real stretch—to look at a cardiogram and say, "This shows evidence that you *will* have a heart attack." Its predictive value is limited.

That said, does it make sense to get one baseline electrocardiogram sometime early in your life, perhaps in your twenties or thirties? Yes, it does, for a very sound and simple reason: It allows you to compare a new cardiogram to an old one. That's one thing doctors look for when they're trying to figure out what's wrong with you—a change in cardiogram findings. Therefore, it's reasonable to have a baseline cardiogram somewhere along the way, preferably before the age of forty. Get it done and keep a copy for yourself. You may need another one someday before you have a surgical procedure or perhaps just because you're not feeling well, so take the old one with you. Believe me, when you present your doctor with a twenty-year-old cardiogram for the purposes of comparison, your doctor may get down on his hands and knees and kiss your feet. He'll be that grateful.

Many times I've had a cardiogram of a patient that looked truly alarming; then I compared the result to an earlier test result and realized it was the same as it was twenty years earlier. Nothing had really changed. Then I was no longer alarmed. My

blood pressure went down. A "normal" cardiogram finding of-
tentimes is what's normal for you, and your normal may be abnormal for somebody else. But do you need an annual cardiogram?
Probably not.

Holter Monitor

The Holter monitor is a small electrocardiogram machine that
you wear. Battery-powered, it records information of the activity
of the heart for a period of twenty-four hours or more. It's designed to detect heart abnormalities over an extended period.
Cardiologists use the Holter monitor because they suspect that
for some people with symptoms of heart disease, or for people
who are reporting symptoms of heart disease, an electrocardiogram done in the office will miss something that happens
overnight or at home. But does everybody need it? No. If you're
complaining of specific symptoms, then you may have a reason
for it. For anyone else, though, it's likely a waste of time.

Electron Beam CT Scan

The electron beam CT scan is an X-ray test designed to detect
calcium in coronary arteries. We've already discussed that the
calcium found in the plaque in coronary arteries is not really
what gives you a heart attack; it's what gives you angina. However, the conceit behind the electron beam test, the calcium test,
is that the two of them keep close company. It is, after all, unusual to find someone with calcium, that is, hard plaque, in his
coronary arteries who doesn't also have soft plaque. So the electron beam CT scan is an indirect way of looking for soft plaque.
The question is, Who needs an electron beam CT scan? Nobody
really knows. It's not nearly as accurate as an angiogram, al-

though it is far less invasive. I don't think at this moment, if you are asymptomatic and have no family history of heart disease, that you really want this thing. There are simply too many questions about its value that remain unanswered.

And that's about it. These are the important noninvasive tests. Beyond them is a clear line of demarcation. On the other side of that line is the angiogram, followed by a series of procedures escalating in risk and discomfort. You shouldn't even be considering an angiogram (and no doctor should be offering you one) unless you have serious symptoms.

You should, if you are an educated consumer, want to know your simple risk factors that are inexpensive to get, are easy to determine, and don't do any harm: specifically, the lipid profile and blood sugar level. And if you want to add a C-reactive protein level test, fine. Still, if you've gotten your laboratory report card back from the doctor, and your marks are good, take a deep breath, and take the self-test that follows, because you still may be surprised by the results.

Remember, the most important question to ask yourself is "What am I going to do with the results?" They shouldn't convince you to ignore your heart. You need to start the program. The only question is when. And so, when you think about it, what the tests that make sense really tell you is how urgent it is to begin controlling your heart attack risk *right now*.

With that in mind, you can evaluate, roughly, your individual risk for heart attack by using the tests recommended in this chapter, and some basic information you already know about yourself. And that's what we're going to do next.

CHAPTER ELEVEN

A Self-test

Here's a self-test to evaluate your risk of heart attack.

Admittedly, this test is pretty crude. A lot of it is based on hard statistical data, some on informed guesswork and common sense. You can choose to skip this chapter entirely and jump right into the program. Take an aspirin a day. Get tested for *Chlamydia pneumoniae* or ask your doctor for a course of antibiotics. Begin statin therapy. I have no problem with anyone who chooses that route, because I think virtually everyone will benefit from it. Still, since any therapy has side effects, and this program is no exception, you may want to know whether you're at low, medium, or high risk for heart attack in the next ten years. It will help you estimate your own risk/benefit ratio.

The point of this chapter is merely to help you estimate whether or not you want to embark upon a journey that will help you prevent your risk of premature death. As I've said from page 1, knowledge is power.

As you go through this test, remember: Honesty is paramount. You can throw the score sheet away when you're through if you don't like your score. So calculate the number and then decide what you are going to do about it.

Body Mass Index

Body mass index is a measure of how much you weigh versus how much you should weigh. It also takes into account your body type, because, as it turns out, your mother was right: There are some people who have "big bones." These people can weigh more and not be "fat." For people who are petite, a small increase in weight can be more of an issue than it would be for somebody else. Body mass index, then, is a way to determine whether or not your weight for your body build is correct, a little too high, or obese. The question really is, Does weight matter? And the answer is, yes, it does.

If you take a look at a lot of the literature, you'll find that, typically, the standard ways to assess your heart disease risk don't address the issue of weight directly; they tiptoe around it. They look at those conditions that weight has been known to affect and then ask about those conditions. For example, they ask about diabetes, they ask about blood pressure, they ask about exercise, knowing full well that people who are too large are more prone to have diabetes, to have high blood pressure, and not to exercise. All that being said, one of the easiest things to do is lump it all together and say, How much do you weigh? Do you weigh too much or not?

We are beginning to learn that there is probably a direct effect of weight on your heart that is not yet well understood. There are some articles now in the literature that support the contention that simply being obese—being seriously overweight—can have a direct effect on your electrocardiogram (ECG). What this effect portends is not clear, but insofar as your

ECG can become abnormal if you get too fat, I don't like it. I think there is some evidence now that weight alone is an independent risk factor, and it certainly predisposes you to other disease states that increase your risk for heart disease. So we're going to go right to the source and ask about weight.

If you look at the table on page 192, you'll see that body mass index can be divided into four groups: normal, overweight, obese, and extremely obese. Calculate your body mass index by locating your height (in inches) and weight on the table. The corresponding number at the top of the table is your body mass index. For example, if you're six feet tall (72 inches) and weigh 191 pounds, your body mass index would be 26: slightly overweight.

If your body mass index falls into the first group on this table (19 to 24), then give yourself a score of 0 point.

If you fall into the second group (25 to 29), give yourself 1 point.

If you fall into the third group (30 to 39), give yourself 5 points.

If your body mass index is above 39, take 10 points.

The reason for this sudden and dramatic 5-point increase for the last group is that research shows that although a little additional weight doesn't greatly increase your risk of heart disease, extreme obesity does. A body mass index greater than 40 places you in dangerous territory.

Body Shape

People have long debated the importance of weight distribution. Does it matter whether you carry excess weight in your waist, as opposed to your upper body? Years ago this question—"Is it better to be shaped like a pear or an apple?"—was dismissed by

BODY MASS INDEX TABLE

	NORMAL						OVERWEIGHT					OBESE										EXTREME OBESITY														
BMI	19	20	21	22	23	24	25	26	27	28	29	30	31	32	33	34	35	36	37	38	39	40	41	42	43	44	45	46	47	48	49	50	51	52	53	54
Height (inches)												**Body Weight (Pounds)**																								
58	91	96	100	105	110	115	119	124	129	134	138	143	148	153	158	162	167	172	177	181	186	191	196	201	205	210	215	220	224	229	234	239	244	248	253	258
59	94	99	104	109	114	119	124	128	133	138	143	148	153	158	163	168	173	178	183	188	193	198	203	208	212	217	222	227	232	237	242	247	252	257	262	267
60	97	102	107	112	118	123	128	133	138	143	148	153	158	163	168	174	179	184	189	194	199	204	209	215	220	225	230	235	240	245	250	255	261	266	271	276
61	100	106	111	116	122	127	132	137	143	148	153	158	164	169	174	180	185	190	195	201	206	211	217	222	227	232	238	243	248	254	259	264	269	275	280	285
62	104	109	115	120	126	131	136	142	147	153	158	164	169	175	180	186	191	196	202	207	213	218	224	229	235	240	246	251	256	262	267	273	278	284	289	295
63	107	113	118	124	130	135	141	146	152	158	163	169	175	180	186	191	197	203	208	214	220	225	231	237	242	248	254	259	265	270	278	282	287	293	299	304
64	110	116	122	128	134	140	145	151	157	163	169	174	180	186	192	197	204	209	215	221	227	232	238	244	250	256	262	267	273	279	285	291	296	302	308	314
65	114	120	126	132	138	144	150	156	162	168	174	180	186	192	198	204	210	216	222	228	234	240	246	252	258	264	270	276	282	288	294	300	306	312	318	324
66	118	124	130	136	142	148	155	161	167	173	179	186	192	198	204	210	216	223	229	235	241	247	253	260	266	272	278	284	291	297	303	309	315	322	328	334
67	121	127	134	140	146	153	159	166	172	178	185	191	198	204	211	217	223	230	236	242	249	255	261	268	274	280	287	293	299	306	312	319	325	331	338	344
68	125	131	138	144	151	158	164	171	177	184	190	197	203	210	216	223	230	236	243	249	256	262	269	276	282	289	295	302	308	315	322	328	335	341	348	354
69	128	135	142	149	155	162	169	176	182	189	196	203	209	216	223	230	236	243	250	257	263	270	277	284	291	297	304	311	318	324	331	338	345	351	358	365
70	132	139	146	153	160	167	174	181	188	195	202	209	216	222	229	236	243	250	257	264	271	278	285	292	299	306	313	320	327	334	341	348	355	362	369	376
71	136	143	150	157	165	172	179	186	193	200	208	215	222	229	236	243	250	257	265	272	279	286	293	301	308	315	322	329	338	343	351	358	365	372	379	386
72	140	147	154	162	169	177	184	191	199	206	213	221	228	235	242	250	258	265	272	279	287	294	302	309	316	324	333	338	346	353	361	368	375	383	390	397
73	144	151	159	166	174	182	189	197	204	212	219	227	235	242	250	257	265	272	280	288	295	302	310	318	325	333	340	348	355	363	371	378	386	393	401	408
74	148	155	163	171	179	186	194	202	210	218	225	233	241	249	256	264	272	280	287	295	303	311	319	326	334	342	350	358	365	373	381	389	396	404	412	420
75	152	160	168	176	184	192	200	208	216	224	232	240	248	256	264	272	279	287	295	303	311	319	327	335	343	351	359	367	375	383	391	399	407	415	423	431
76	156	164	172	180	189	197	205	213	221	230	238	246	254	263	271	279	287	295	304	312	320	328	336	344	353	361	369	377	385	394	402	410	418	426	435	443

Source: Adapted from Clinical Guidelines in the Identification, Evaluation, and Treatment of Overweight and Obesity in Adults: The Evidence Report.

doctors as so much grocery-store, diet-book, self-help nonsense. What possible difference could it make whether your fat was located in your waist or your elbows? Surprisingly enough, it does matter. There is indeed a difference between trunkal fat—fat located around your waist and abdomen—and fat found elsewhere in your body. Simply put: If you have a big waist, you have a problem.

So get out the tape measure and calculate your waist size. Don't hold your breath. Don't cheat. Just relax and take an honest measurement. If you're a male and the circumference of your waist exceeds forty inches, give yourself 1 point. If it's forty inches or less, give yourself 0 point. For women, the magic number is thirty-five. Beyond that number, you get 1 point.

Age

Clearly, as you grow older, the risk of getting a heart attack in the ensuing ten years goes up. People who are twenty years old have not had enough time for development of heart disease, so their risk of getting heart disease in the next ten years is low. As you age, the risk increases. It's as simple as that. Age, all by itself, is a marker for heart disease, so determining your score on this question is as simple as knowing your age.

- **20 TO 39**—Statistically, the odds for developing heart disease are quite low. Give yourself 0 point.
- **40–54**—Unfortunately, matters change pretty dramatically as you enter middle age. Give yourself 12 points if you fall into this category. There is nothing you can do about it.
- **55 AND OVER**—Sorry; fasten your seat belt and give yourself 25 points.

Tobacco

The use of tobacco, in any form, is an enormous health risk. For the purposes of this test, however, we're talking strictly about smoking, which is a very dangerous thing to do.

On this, everyone in the medical community is in agreement. Stop! Now! It doesn't matter that we don't really know why smoking leads to heart disease. Although one explanation, as we've discussed, is that it predisposes you to *C. pneumoniae*, which should make you predisposed to having a heart attack. Have we nailed this down for sure? No, but it's as good an explanation as we have. And that is the overriding theme of this book: I am recommending some actions without necessarily understanding the mechanism behind their benefits. So, ask yourself the question: Do you smoke or don't you? (I'll admit this sounds a bit like Clint Eastwood: "Do you feel lucky today, or not?" At least one guy in the movie got his head blown off answering that question wrong.)

If you don't smoke, pat yourself on the head and give yourself 0 point.

If you are smoking, give yourself 10 points, pat yourself somewhere else—hard!—and throw away your cigarettes. Please!

Complicating this question is the issue of quitting. What if you're a former smoker? A good and fair question, and one without an easy answer. For the purposes of this book, what I'm going to do is give you a pass. Congratulations! Just don't ever start smoking again. Truthfully, it's very hard to know what to do with ex-smokers from a statistical standpoint. I can't tell you how many times I've wheeled someone to the operating room after he's suffered a heart attack and endured the following exchange:

"Do you smoke?"

"No?"

"When did you quit?"

"This morning."

So answer the question honestly. If you just quit this morning, when you bought this book, then you're a smoker. If you quit two weeks ago, and you're hoping you can stay off, but you can still feel the craving deep in your soul, then you're a smoker. If, however, you quit five years ago, I'm willing to give you a break. You've earned it.

Blood pressure

Since blood pressure changes from day to day, minute to minute, no single measurement is adequate. My recommendation is that you check your blood pressure three or four times over the course of a week or two and then compute the average. A caveat: Clearly, if the first measurement is astronomically high, do it again quickly, and then go see the doctor, but if it's normal— roughly 120 (systolic) over 80 (diastolic)—then do it a few more times and see where it sits. If you're wondering whether those shopping mall blood pressure machines work, the surprising answer seems to be that they do. In fact, because people tend to get nervous in a doctor's office, doctors' office blood pressures may be artificially high. They are expensive, too.

For the purposes of this test, we're going to look specifically at the systolic reading. If that number is below 120, give yourself 0 points. If it's between 120 and 160, you get 4 points. If it's greater than 160, give yourself 8 points.

The reason this is important should be pretty clear. Think about the term *blood pressure*. What does it mean? Well, it's exactly what it appears to be: the amount of pressure the heart is generating with every beat. That's the systolic number, which reflects how hard the heart is pumping. So if it's pumping harder, it's using more oxygen; it's hungrier, and it's going to be at higher risk of getting into trouble. (By the way, we're talking about how hard your heart is working during normal use, not during exercise, which is another issue entirely; the heart is supposed to work harder during exercise.)

Now, what if you're in that low or middle range primarily because you're on blood pressure medication? Again, for the purposes of this test, I'll give you a pass. Your blood pressure is under control. That's what matters most. But you are not absolved of the requirement to keep your blood pressure low. Statins, aspirin, and antibiotics are not a substitute for your blood pressure pills.

Genetics

Take a close look at your family tree. Is there a history of heart disease, in particular, heart attack? If your close blood relatives—mother, father, siblings, grandparents, aunts, uncles, anyone within two degrees of separation—have had heart disease or heart attack, you should be concerned. Of course, one incident does not a pattern make; we're looking for a trend here.

So, for the sake of this test, let's use the number 2. If two or more people in your immediate family (as defined here) have had significant coronary events (this includes heart attack, angioplasty, bypass surgery), give yourself 4 points. If not, you get 0 point.

The explanation is simple: Heart attacks run in families. If your grandfather and father both dropped dead of a massive heart attack at fifty-five, and you're fifty-four, you have reason to be anxious.

Diabetes

Diabetes includes all kinds of diabetes: juvenile-onset, insulin-dependent diabetes, diabetes you treat with diet alone, diabetes treated with medication. If you hear the word *diabetes* linked with "you" in your doctor's office, you are at increased risk. The reason is that diabetes is strongly associated with vascular disease. We know that diabetics get heart disease at an accelerated rate, we know they get it younger, and we know that when they have heart attacks, their heart attacks are more severe. Every way you look at diabetes, it's bad for your heart.

So, if you have diabetes, give yourself 8 points; if not, 0.

Ah, but what if you are successfully managing your diabetes with medication? Does that reduce your risk, in much the same way that treating high blood pressure with medication reduces risk? In other words, shouldn't you get 0 point if your diabetes is under control? The answer is no. The presence of diabetes, by itself, is enough to make you a permanent 8-point candidate. Why? I don't know. And nobody else does either.

Cholesterol

In order to complete this portion of the test, you'll have to get a cholesterol test. If, for some reason, you don't want a test, then the only safe thing for you to do is max out on all these questions. Really though, the only way to gauge your heart attack risk accurately is to know your cholesterol level. And for the most accurate picture, you should know all three of the important numbers. I'm talking about HDL, LDL, and triglyceride levels—the big three! Together, these three numbers paint a portrait of your blood lipids and allow you to know just how much work you need to do.

LDL CHOLESTEROL

This is the bad cholesterol: you don't want much of it in your blood. If your blood test reveals an LDL reading of less than 100, give yourself 0 points. If it's between 100 and 190, give yourself 10 points. If it's above 190, give yourself 20 points, and then call your doctor!

HDL CHOLESTEROL

The good cholesterol: if your reading is above 55, give yourself 0 points. If it's between 36 and 54, give yourself 5 points. If it's 35 or below, add 10 points.

TRIGLYCERIDES

Triglycerides are tiny particles of fat found in your blood. As with LDL, too much is a very bad thing. So if your triglyceride reading is less than 100, give yourself 0 points. If it's between 100 and 199, give yourself 2 points. If it's greater than 200, add 4 points.

Bonus Question

Do you drink alcohol? There is a growing body of evidence to suggest that moderate use of alcohol, and by *moderate* I mean one to two drinks per day, at most, offers some protection against heart disease. Whereas once we thought that only red wine offered this benefit, more recent research indicates that the agent of protection may in fact be the alcohol itself. So it really doesn't matter what you drink, so long as you consume it in moderation. Therefore, if you consume one to two drinks per day, *subtract* 2 points from your total score. If you don't drink at all, or only rarely, you get no bonus. (If you consume more than two alcoholic beverages per day, well, you've got other problems, and you probably should be reading a different book.) And there you are. That's the test. Now add up your points. (Remember, these are just ballpark figures, but they will give you some idea of where you stand in the battle against heart disease.)

0 TO 32 POINTS—Low risk: If you fall in this range, congratulations. Your risk of having a coronary event in the next ten years is probably 3 percent or less.

33 TO 56 POINTS—Medium risk: If you fall in this range, your risk of having a coronary event in the next ten years is somewhere between 3 and 10 percent.

67 POINTS OR ABOVE—High risk: If you fall in this range, you have reason to be extremely concerned. Your risk of having a coronary event in the next ten years is at least 10 percent, and perhaps as high as 30 percent.

The problem with statistics is that it's difficult to know what they mean for any individual. Follow a large group of people for ten years, add up the points for each of its members, and you will find that they "sort out" predictably. The high-risk group will have more deaths due to heart disease. The low-risk groups will have fewer. This makes statisticians happy. But clinicians, who deal with individual patients, and the patients themselves, are a different matter. They don't want to know how many of a group will die. The clinicians and the patients ask a different question: "How do these numbers apply to an individual?" Or "Am I going to die of a heart attack tomorrow?" Sorry, but nobody knows that answer. The "point system" answers the question only indirectly. That's not very satisfying, but it's the best answer anyone can give right now.

If you are in a high-risk group, you need to be worried about imminent heart attack and death. You need to take immediate action to modify those risk factors that you can. You need to see a doctor right away. And you should begin the statin-aspirin-antibiotic program.

The middle group may have more time to think it over, but it's not a terrific group to be in either. Here again the risk of death from heart attack exceeds the risk of the prevention program. Go for it.

If you're in the low-risk group you face some fascinating and subtle questions. Your risk of having a heart attack in the next ten years is pretty low, although it is not zero. There are risks to the program. That might prompt you to say, "I'll worry about all this tomorrow." But that's like Wimpy in the Popeye comics saying, "I'll gladly pay you Tuesday for a hamburger today." Eventually Wimpy's burger tab is going to catch up with him. The same is true of your heart disease tab. Damage builds on damage. You may, in the end, pay your heart disease tab with your life. It is much better in my opinion to turn off the disease process early and keep things in the walls of your coronary arteries quiet than to dive in later and try to patch up those walls. Here, too, the advice I have is straightforward. You are better off on the program than off it.

Again, after all the risk analysis, the message is clear. The great majority of people should be taking statins, aspirin, and a course of antibiotics.

HEART ATTACK RISK SCORE SHEET		POINTS	TOTAL
1. WEIGHT: BMI	19-25	0	
	26–30	1	
	31–40	5	
	>40	10	
2. SHAPE	Apple	0	
	Pear	1	
3. AGE	20-39	0	
	40–54	12	
	>55	25	
4. TOBACCO USE	No	0	
	Yes	10	
5. SYSTOLIC BLOOD PRESSURE	<120	0	
	120–160	4	
	>160	8	
6. FAMILY HISTORY OF HEART DISEASE	No	0	
	Yes	4	
7. DIABETES	No	0	
	Yes	8	
8. LDL CHOLESTEROL	<100	0	
	100–190	10	
	>190	20	
9. HDL CHOLESTEROL	<35	10	
	36–54	5	
	>54	0	
10. TRIGLYCERIDES	<100	0	
	100–199	2	
	>199	4	
11. BONUS QUESTION ALCOHOL	N	0	
	Y*	-2	

*No more than 2 drinks/day

CHAPTER TWELVE

The Eldest Brother

The eldest brother in the Chinese parable was brilliant enough to realize that the true business of the healing arts is improving the public health. You can do this one person at a time. But it is far better, not to mention cheaper for society at large, to change the environment in which we live and make it safer.

That is what this book is all about. It is the stuff of the eldest brother. We have seen the conditions that predispose all of us to heart attack and premature death. We have seen what must be done to change those conditions. Now we must do those things that must be done.

On an individual level you can change the way you live and you can "get with the program." I think it is a sensible way to keep yourself alive longer, and to live better. You can tell your friends about the program and help them to live better, too. The more people who read this book and follow its advice, the more I will have accomplished my goal as a doctor by improving the health of all around me.

But society can do better than that. We have it in our power to make public health policy that will help millions of people who may never read or hear of this book. We can change the way we regulate the medications that can save lives, and that includes statins. In fact, we should not be "prescribing" statins at all. Statins should be available over the counter.

What are the objections to deregulating statins? First, the critics will point to the "liver function abnormalities" that occasionally show up in statin users. These abnormal blood test results rarely result in clinical disease. In the September 15, 2002, issue of the *American Journal of Cardiology* (vol. 90, no. 6), editor in chief William Clifford Roberts, M.D., cites an amazing statistic: The rate of acute liver failure produced by statins is one case for every 1 million patient-treatment years. This is about equal to the rate of spontaneous liver failure in America—that is, liver failure that just happens, out of the blue, with no identifiable cause. Dr. Roberts sums up matters pretty well when he says, "The danger for a patient with an elevated serum LDL cholesterol is arterial, not hepatic!" (The exclamation point is his, not mine.) If you're even more curious, check out the article by Keith G. Tolman, "The liver and lovastatin" in the *American Journal of Cardiology* (June 15, 2002, vol. 89, pp. 1374–80).

The critics will also talk about the muscle disease that some statin users experience, statin myopathy. In severe cases this problem can lead to kidney failure, and even death. The statin that caused truly ferocious muscle problems, Baycol, is no longer on the market. Baycol wreaked havoc as a prescription drug, not over the counter, by the way. The other statins have much safer muscle-risk profiles. Statin myopathy occurs in about 1 in 10,000 person-years (again check Dr. Roberts's article for more details and an article by Carlos A. Dujovne, M.D., in the June 15, 2002, issue of the *American Journal of Cardiology*, vol. 89, no. 12, pp. 1411–13). There's a lot of math to look at if you really want to do so, but the bottom line is simple: You're more likely to have a major aspirin bleed than experience statin myopathy. What's more, the muscle abnormalities they produce usually cause symptoms. You can often tell that the drug is giving you trouble and you can stop taking it.

We have experience with an over-the-counter statin, Cholestin, which has not seemed to cause much trouble at all. And Cholestin is relatively unregulated. There is no guarantee of its purity or consistency from one dosage to the next. If pharmaceutical-grade statins were available over the counter, we would all feel more comfortable that the dosages we were taking were precisely the doses we wanted (and the dosages the bottle said we were taking).

There are plenty of sane cardiologists and public health experts who joke about putting a "shaker" of statin on the table of every steak restaurant in America. The interesting thing is, they're not really joking. Most of them believe it would do a lot of good. I agree, except that I think we should expand the recommendation to every table of every restaurant in America. And it should be in every home, too.

The best way to achieve this end is not with a "statin-shaker" but with a supply of easily obtained, over-the-counter statins available in drugstores, groceries, and convenience stores everywhere.

The aspirin issue is different. Aspirin is already available over the counter. The only question is who should be taking it. Critics will point to the potential for bleeding if everybody takes an aspirin a day. They have a point. But look at the record. Millions of people take aspirin in this country every day. A few have trouble. Most do not. Those with a history of bleeding should have that problem looked at by a doctor before they embark upon a lifetime of aspirin therapy. But that is true for them if they take even a short course of aspirin for a headache or a common cold. Again, the researchers are taking a close look at the old saw "People with ulcers must never take aspirin," and they are finding that the truth is not nearly as absolute as the statement implies.

Some people have ulcers and need them treated. For some of them *H. pylori* needs to be eradicated. Others have small bleeds from other clearly identifiable sources that can be corrected. Once these folks have their problems addressed, aspirin is probably safe for them. More recent papers suggest that the blood loss people suffer from taking an aspirin a day tends to be negligible.

ICU docs with their draconian view of disease usually say, "Go ahead and bleed; we can fix that. But don't have a heart attack because that damage is permanent." This attitude ignores the problem that people who bleed enough to become anemic often have heart attacks as a result. The recent literature is far more encouraging. It says, "Go ahead and take an aspirin a day; the odds are you won't bleed significantly enough to give you trouble."

The suggestion that we need to recommend even wider use of antibiotics makes a lot of people angry. Don't suggest this to your friend, the infectious disease expert, over dinner. You may have to perform the Heimlich maneuver. But if you get past the shock of the initial suggestion and discuss a program that would save lives, you will often find that even the most conservative doctors can think of a program that will keep the nation safe from "superbugs." Perhaps we need a national heart antibiotic policy. This would rotate the antichlamydial antibiotics we use each month. January might be "antibiotic A" month, February "antibiotic B" month, and so on. This would keep the bacteria off balance and prevent them from becoming resistant to any particular drug. We do this in the hospital all the time. I usually have to ask my infectious disease colleagues, "Which prophylactic antibiotics are we using on any given day for our heart patients?" because they are trying to stay one step ahead of the bacteria.

This plan would require a national antibiotic information center and a national antibiotic coordinating committee. But we have organized much larger projects in the past. Any nation that can come together and coordinate a Hoover Dam, or the distribution of polio vaccine (not to mention the simultaneous distribution of millions of copies of Harry Potter books on the day they are published) should be able to handle this relatively minor program.

Assuming we do what needs to be done and make statins available, increase our use of aspirin, and give more antibiotics to people, what will be the impact of the program? The simple answer is that there will be many fewer deaths from heart attacks among relatively young people. Of course, we will have to redefine *young*. Perhaps, if the heart attack rate drops precipitously, "young people" will be folks in their sixties. And this is not an idle distinction.

I was discussing this plan with a doctor friend, who suddenly said, "Good grief! If this program works, I'm going to outlive my 401K plan!"

He was joking. But his comment carries real import. As people live longer, society is going to have to adjust to care for them. Retirement plan calculations will be inaccurate. Insurance company "life tables" will slowly become unreliable. An aging population will continue to require health care long after their budgeted allotment from the Medicare folks will have run dry. Medicare is in trouble now as the baby boomers (that's me, by the way) age into the beneficiary group. What will happen as these aging Americans refuse to die on schedule is anybody's guess.

America's health care delivery system will have to find innovative ways to pay for the care that more, older citizens will require. The pessimists among us raise the specter of the *R* word, *rationing*, to accommodate the elderly. Americans have never been very comfortable with that concept, and they probably won't be in the future. No doubt about it: Longer lifetimes are going to create problems for people in authority.

So be it. You shouldn't have to die because someone's tax rates might go up. You shouldn't agree to rust out to preserve the Medicare trust fund. And you deserve to live well into your older years despite the fact that you will have more of those years than the pencil pushers and bean counters planned on. It's going to get complicated, no doubt about it. So the time to start thinking about solutions to these and other problems is now, not ten years from now.

The journey to a healthier America is a long one. It has just begun. But we can't despair over its length, nor its tortuous course.

The *Tao Te Ching* (on which was based our ancient Chinese parable) has one other piece of advice that we would all do well to remember:

"A journey of a thousand miles begins with a single step."

Afterword: The Pace of Progress

■ ■ ■

As soon as I finished typing the Bibliography, more fascinating articles appeared. They are a signal that matters are heating up in the "inflammation and heart disease" arena among the traditional journals. That's good, because most of the time, as we've discussed, the pace of progress can be maddeningly slow.

New medicine can take a long time to get to you, the person who needs it. If you wait for new stuff to percolate through official channels, you can literally die waiting.

The basic research alone can take decades to achieve results. When a new treatment or concept is about to make an impact, articles about it bubble to the surface in the "big journals." You've probably heard of some of them. They include the *British Medical Journal (BMJ)*, *The Lancet*, the *Journal of the American Medical Association (JAMA)*, *Circulation*, and, of course, the grandaddy of them all, the *New England Journal of Medicine (N Engl J Med)*.

The editors at the *NEJM* are quite picky about what they print. And they are ferociously protective of their priority. If they're going to publish your work, they want to be its exclusive source. Woe unto the prospective author who leaks stories about his or her work to the press before the *Journal* has published it. So it's not surprising that until the *NEJM* has either published a study, or passed on it, you're not likely to see much about the research in the popular press.

But once the *New England Journal* (or one of the other "big journals") has given its imprimatur to something, the popular press begins to print bits and pieces of what's going on. This is when most people catch wind of something new. Unfortunately, the coverage of medical progress from that point forward becomes haphazard and often unreliable. Watching the popular press grapple with medical stories has become a parlor game among physicians. Who got the science right? Who inflated its significance out of all proportion? Who played medicine as tabloid news, and who took the time and column inches to put the story into perspective?

It's not surprising that some news sources are better than others. The *New York Times*, in particular, has a terrific group of medical journalists. Several of the television networks have M.D.'s reporting on medicine. All this publicity begins to accelerate the adoption process. For one thing, patients start walking into their doctor's office and asking questions. That often sends the docs scurrying to look things up.

The FDA needs to get involved at some point if the new drugs need approval, or if the new techniques need to be evaluated. Then "thought leaders" in medicine begin to go about publishing position papers. These are statements from the medical bureaucracy that establish official opinions on the new development. This gives physicians the official green light to offer the new drugs, or new treatments, to patients (some doctors don't wait for position papers, of course; they adopt early and wait for everyone else to catch up).

All the while, people who might have benefited from the new treatments are waiting. This waiting makes sense if the new treatments are dangerous, or if the diseases they treat are not lethal. But it makes little sense if the treatments are not particularly harmful, or if the patients waiting to try the treatments are dying.

The process, from start to finish, can take dozens of years. So the question we need to answer is, Where are we, in the traditional adoption process, regarding the new treatments outlined in this book?

Take a look at the Bibliography with an educated eye, and you can spot lots of articles from the high-profile journals. There are position papers in there, too. These articles are typically narrow in scope. They don't often link up with articles from other specialties. They're making recommendations, and they're making the news, but in bits and pieces.

What has been missing is the grand synthesis that our program offers. Conditions are beginning to change, though. The staid, conservative medical literature is beginning to catch up to this book.

The *British Medical Journal* (June 28, 2003) published a series of three papers and an accompanying editorial. Two of the articles carried the shocking (by medical journal standards, anyway) titles "A strategy to reduce cardiovascular disease by more than 80%" and "A cure for cardiovascular disease?" As if that weren't striking enough, the editorial noted what it called one of the boldest claims for a new intervention—"a greater impact on the prevention of disease in the Western world than any other known intervention."

What was the intervention? It was what the authors called a "Polypill," which combined a statin and aspirin with other drugs. The authors were ecstatic. They filed for a patent on the pill's formulation and applied for a trademark on the name *Polypill*.

This implies that the pace of change is accelerating. You can expect organized medicine to begin recommending the program in this book sooner rather than later. How soon? Within the next five years or so, if history is any guide. Watch the press and you'll see this whole topic heating up to a fever pitch.

But you don't have to wait five years. This book has put you way ahead of the curve. You know about statins. You know about aspirin. You know about *Chlamydia pneumoniae*, too, which the *BMJ* authors didn't address. You don't need to wait for a Polypill or an official position paper. Every day you wait to start the program in this book is another lost opportunity to turn off the heart disease process.

Let others wait for official bureaucratic approval; you can begin saving your own life right now.

Bibliography

■ ■ ■

The sheer volume of material written about heart disease is overwhelming. There are thousands of journal articles, textbook chapters, newspaper and magazine citations, all of them adding to what we know about America's leading killer.

If you're interested in reading more about the program, I've listed some of the source material used to compile this book. The list is not complete by any means. It is not the last word on any of the subjects we've discussed either. As soon as I finish typing this page, I'm certain that more articles will become available.

I have divided the articles into rather broad catagories. Even so, there is a lot of overlap. An article dealing with the effect of statins on C-reactive protein, for example, could have been placed with either the statin group or the C-reactive protein group.

Some of these articles are pretty dense; others are more accessible. Most of them are fun to explore.

ASPIRIN

Aronow WS. Thrombolysis and antithrombotic therapy for coronary artery disease. *Clin Geriatr Med* 2001; 17(1):173–188.

Aspirin. In: Nissen D, editor. *Mosby's drug consult*. St. Louis: Mosby, Inc., 2002; 212–230.

Catella-Lawson F. Vascular biology of thrombosis: platelet-vessel wall interactions and aspirin effects. *Neurology* 2001; 57(5 Suppl 2):S5–S7.

Greenberg PD, Cello JP, Rockey DC. Relationship of low-dose aspirin to GI injury and occult bleeding: a pilot study. *Gastrointest Endosc* 1999; 50(5):618–622.

Hawkey CJ, Lanas AI. Doubt and certainty about nonsteroidal anti-inflammatory drugs in the year 2000: a multidisciplinary expert statement. *Am J Med* 2001; 110(1A):79S–100S.

Miser WF. An aspirin a day keeps the MI away (for some). *Am Fam Physician* 2002; 65(10):2000, 2003.

Mukamal KJ, Mittleman MA, Maclure M, Sherwood JB, Goldberg RJ, Muller JE. Recent aspirin use is associated with smaller myocardial infarct size and lower likelihood of Q-wave infarction. *Am Heart J* 1999; 137(6): 1120–1128.

Newby LK, Califf RM, White HD, Harrington RA, Van de WF, Granger CB et al. The failure of orally administered glycoprotein IIb/IIIa inhibitors to prevent recurrent cardiac events. *Am J Med* 2002; 112(8):647–658.

Ray WA, Murray KT. Aspirin: redundant in users of nonaspirin, nonsteroidal antiinflammatory agents? *Am Heart J* 2002; 143(3):381–382.

Shah PK. Plaque disruption and thrombosis. Potential role of inflammation and infection. *Cardiol Clin* 1999; 17(2):271–281.

U.S. Preventative Services Task Force. Aspirin for the primary prevention of cardiovascular events: recommendations and rationale. *Am Fam Physician* 2002; 65(10):2107–2110.

Verheugt FW, Gersh BJ. Aspirin beyond platelet inhibition. *Am J Cardiol* 2002; 90(1):39–41.

Weissmann G. NSAIDS: aspirin and aspirin-like drugs. In: Goldman L, Bennett JC, editors. *Cecil textbook of medicine*. Philadelphia: W.B. Saunders, 2000; 114–118.

BODY WEIGHT

Aronne LJ. Obesity and weight gain. In: Noble J, Green HL, editors. *Textbook of primary care medicine*. St. Louis: Mosby, 2001; 486–491.

Corbi GM, Carbone S, Ziccardi P, Giugliano G, Marfella R, Nappo F et al. FFAs and QT intervals in obese women with visceral adiposity: effects of sustained weight loss over 1 year. *J Clin Endocrinol Metab* 2002; 87(5): 2080–2083.

Fahey PJ, Wood JC. Obesity and Lipids. *Clinics in Family Practice* 2000; 2(2).

Hyder ML, O'Byrne KK, Poston WSC, Foreyt JP. Behavior modification in the treatment of obesity. *Clinics in Family Practice* 2002; 4(2).

Kannel WB, Wilson PW, Nam BH, D'Agostino RB. Risk stratification of obesity as a coronary risk factor. *Am J Cardiol* 2002; 90(7): 697–701.

Landi F, Zuccala G, Gambassi G, Incalzi RA, Manigrasso L, Pagano F et al. Body mass index and mortality among older people living in the community. *J Am Geriatr Soc* 1999; 47(9):1072–1076.

Mauriege P, Brochu M, Prud'homme D, Tremblay A, Nadeau A, Lemieux S et al. Is visceral adiposity a significant correlate of subcutaneous adipose cell lipolysis in men? *J Clin Endocrinol Metab* 1999; 84(2):736–742.

Purnell JQ, Kahn SE, Albers JJ, Nevin DN, Brunzell JD, Schwartz RS. Effect of weight loss with reduction of intra-abdominal fat on lipid metabolism in older men. *J Clin Endocrinol Metab* 2000; 85(3):977–982.

Rea TD, Heckbert SR, Kaplan RC, Psaty BM, Smith NL, Lemaitre RN et al. Body mass index and the risk of recurrent coronary events following acute myocardial infarction. *Am J Cardiol* 2001; 88(5):467–472.

Rosengren A. Improved diet and lifestyle in middle-aged women helped reduce the incidence of CHD: A combination of diet, exercise, alcohol consumption, body-mass index and non-smoking status is associated with a very low risk of CHD among women. *Evidence-based Cardiovascular Medicine* 2000; 4(4):92–94.

Vega GL. Results of Expert Meetings: Obesity and Cardiovascular Disease. Obesity, the metabolic syndrome, and cardiovascular disease. *Am Heart J* 2001; 142(6):1108–1116.

REACTIVE PROTEIN

Albert MA, Danielson E, Rifai N, Ridker PM. Effect of statin therapy on C-reactive protein levels: the pravastatin inflammation/CRP evaluation (PRINCE): a randomized trial and cohort study. *JAMA* 2001; 286(1):64–70.

Bays HE, Stein EA, Shah AK, Maccubbin DL, Mitchel YB, Mercuri M. Effects of simvastatin on C-reactive protein in mixed hyperlipidemic and hyper-triglyceridemic patients. *Am J Cardiol* 2002; 90(9):942–946.

Bickel C, Rupprecht HJ, Blankenberg S, Espiniola-Klein C, Schlitt A, Rippin G et al. Relation of markers of inflammation (C-reactive protein, fibrinogen, von Willebrand factor, and leukocyte count) and statin therapy to long-term mortality in patients with angiographically proven coronary artery disease. *Am J Cardiol* 2002; 89(8):901–908.

Emery G. Protein may be good heart attack predictor—study. Reuters News 2002 Nov 13.

Folsom AR, Aleksic N, Catellier D, Juneja HS, Wu KK. C-reactive protein and incident coronary heart disease in the Atherosclerosis Risk In Communities (ARIC) study. *Am Heart J* 2002; 144(2):233–238.

Folsom AR, Pankow JS, Tracy RP, Arnett DK, Peacock JM, Hong Y et al. Association of C-reactive protein with markers of prevalent atherosclerotic disease. *Am J Cardiol* 2001; 88(2):112–117.

Grady D. Study says a protein may be better than cholesterol in predicting heart disease risk. *New York Times* 2002 Nov 14;A26.

Libby P, Ridker PM. Novel inflammatory markers of coronary risk: theory versus practice. *Circulation* 1999; 100(11):1148–1150.

Ridker PM, Rifai N, Clearfield M, Downs JR, Weis SE, Miles JS et al. Measurement of C-reactive protein for the targeting of statin therapy in the primary prevention of acute coronary events. *N Engl J Med* 2001; 344(26): 1959–1965.

Ridker PM, Rifai N, Rose L, Buring JE, Cook NR. Comparison of C-reactive protein and low-density lipoprotein cholesterol levels in the prediction of first cardiovascular events. *N Engl J Med* 2002; 347(20): 1557–1565.

Speidl WS, Graf S, Hornykewycz S, Nikfardjam M, Niessner A, Zorn G et al. High-sensitivity C-reactive protein in the prediction of coronary events in patients with premature coronary artery disease. *Am Heart J* 2002; 144(3):449–455.

Zebrack JS, Anderson JL, Maycock CA, Horne BD, Bair TL, Muhlestein JB. Usefulness of high-sensitivity C-reactive protein in predicting long-term risk of death or acute myocardial infarction in patients with unstable or stable angina pectoris or acute myocardial infarction. *Am J Cardiol* 2002; 89(2):145–149.

CHOLESTEROL

Albert MA, Staggers J, Chew P, Ridker PM. The pravastatin inflammation CRP evaluation (PRINCE): rationale and design. *Am Heart J* 2001; 141(6): 893–898.

Ansell BJ. Developing a clinical strategy for cholesterol management in an era of unanswered questions. *Am J Cardiol* 2001; 88(4 Suppl):25F–30F.

Ansell BJ, Waters DD. Reassessment of National Cholesterol Education Program Adult Treatment Panel-III guidelines: one year later. *Am J Cardiol* 2002; 90(5): 524–525.

Ballantyne CM. Hyperlipoproteinemias. In: *Conn's current therapy.* Philadelphia: WB Saunders, 2002; 572–577.

Crouch MA. Effective use of statins to prevent coronary heart disease. *Am Fam Physician* 2001; 63(2):309–304.

Davidson MH. A look to the future: new treatment guidelines and a perspective on statins. *Am J Med* 2002; 112 (Suppl 8A):34S–41S.

Fathi R, Haluska B, Short L, Marwick TH. A randomized trial of aggressive lipid reduction for improvement of myocardial ischemia, symptom status, and vascular function in patients with coronary artery disease not amenable to intervention. *Am J Med* 2003; 114(6):445–453.

Fodor JG, Frohlich JJ, Genest JJ, Jr., McPherson PR. Recommendations for the management and treatment of dyslipidemia. Report of the Working Group on Hypercholesterolemia and Other Dyslipidemias. *CMAJ* 2000; 162(10): 1441–1447.

Gillett ER. Hyperlipid treatment options. *Clinics in Family Practice* 2002; 4(3).

Henkel J. Keeping cholesterol under control. *FDA Consum* 1999; 33(1):23–27.

Kornitzer M. Cholesterol lowering primary prevention trials exclude a significant proportion of the general population. *Evidence-based Cardiovascular Medicine* 2001; 5(3):76–77.

Nissen SE. Who is at risk for atherosclerotic disease? Lessons from intravascular ultrasound. *Am J Med* 2002; 112 (Suppl 8A):27S–33S.

Palinski W, Tsimikas S. Immunomodulatory effects of statins: mechanisms and potential impact on arteriosclerosis. *J Am Soc Nephrol* 2002; 13(6): 1673–1681.

Robins SJ. Targeting low high-density lipoprotein cholesterol for therapy: lessons from the Veterans Affairs High-density Lipoprotein Intervention Trial. *Am J Cardiol* 2001; 88(12A):19N–23N.

Rosenson RS. The rationale for combination therapy. *Am J Cardiol* 2002; 90(10B):2K–7K.

Waters DD. Are we aggressive enough in lowering cholesterol? *Am J Cardiol* 2001; 88(4 Suppl):10F–15F.

Zoler ML. Pravastin reduces c-reactive protein levels in large study. *Today in Medicine* 2001 May 24.

DIETS

Atkins RC. *Dr. Atkins' new diet revolution*. New York: M. Evans, 1992.

Foster GD, Wyatt HR, Hill JO, McGuckin BG, Brill C, Mohammed BS et al. A randomized trial of a low-carbohydrate diet for obesity. *N Engl J Med* 2003; 348(21):2082–2090.

Ornish D. *Stress, diet, and your heart*. New York: Holt, Rinehart, and Winston, 1983.

Samaha FF, Iqbal N, Seshadri P, Chicano KL, Daily DA, McGrory J et al. A low-carbohydrate as compared with a low-fat diet in severe obesity. *N Engl J Med* 2003; 348(21):2074–2081.

Schaefer EJ, Augustin JL, McNamara JR, Seman LJ, Bourdet KL, Meydani MM et al. Lipid lowering and weight reduction by home-delivered dietary modification in coronary heart disease patients taking statins. *Am J Cardiol* 2001; 87(8):1000–1003.

Stone NJ, Kushner R. Effects of dietary modification and treatment of obesity. Emphasis on improving vascular outcomes. *Med Clin North Am* 2000; 84(1):95–122.

FITNESS AND EXERCISE

Ades PA, Coello CE. Effects of exercise and cardiac rehabilitation on cardiovascular outcomes. *Med Clin North Am* 2000; 84(1):251–265, x–xi.

Bielak KM, Merket RM. Exercise. *Clinics in Family Practice* 2000; 2(2).

Durstine JL, Thompson PD. Exercise in the treatment of lipid disorders. *Cardiol Clin* 2001; 19(3):471–488.

Katzel LI, Sorkin JD, Goldberg AP. Exercise-induced silent myocardial ischemia and future cardiac events in healthy, sedentary, middle-aged and older men. *J Am Geriatr Soc* 1999; 47(8):923–929.

Kokkinos PF, Choucair W, Graves P, Papademetriou V, Ellahham S. Chronic heart failure and exercise. *Am Heart J* 2000; 140(1):21–28.

Kullo IJ, Hensrud DD, Allison TG. Relation of low cardiorespiratory fitness to the metabolic syndrome in middle-aged men. *Am J Cardiol* 2002; 90(7):795–797.

Lucini D, Milani RV, Costantino G, Lavie CJ, Porta A, Pagani M. Effects of cardiac rehabilitation and exercise training on autonomic regulation in patients with coronary artery disease. *Am Heart J* 2002; 143(6):977–983.

MacKnight JM. Exercise considerations in hypertension, obesity, and dyslipidemia. *Clin Sports Med* 2003; 22(1):101–121, vii.

Myers J, Gianrossi R, Schwitter J, Wagner D, Dubach P. Effect of exercise training on postexercise oxygen uptake kinetics in patients with reduced ventricular function. *Chest* 2001; 120(4):1206–1211.

Myers J, Goebbels U, Dzeikan G, Froelicher V, Bremerich J, Mueller P et al. Exercise training and myocardial remodeling in patients with reduced ventricular function: one-year follow-up with magnetic resonance imaging. *Am Heart J* 2000; 139(2 Pt 1):252–261.

Rivet C. What type of exercise prevents cardiovascular disease in postmenopausal women? *CMAJ* 2003; 168(3):314.

GENERAL PRINCIPLES

Abdelmouttaleb I, Danchin N, Ilardo C, Aimone-Gastin I, Angioi M, Lozniewski A et al. C-Reactive protein and coronary artery disease: additional evidence of the implication of an inflammatory process in acute coronary syndromes. *Am Heart J* 1999; 137(2):346–351.

Ades PA, Coello CE. Effects of exercise and cardiac rehabilitation on cardiovascular outcomes. *Med Clin North Am* 2000; 84(1):251–265, x–xi.

Assmann G, Cullen P, Schulte H. Simple scoring scheme for calculating the risk of acute coronary events based on the 10-year follow-up of the prospective cardiovascular Munster (PROCAM) study. *Circulation* 2002; 105(3): 310–315.

Braunwald E. *Heart disease: a textbook of cardiovascular medicine.* 6th ed. Philadelphia: Saunders, 2001.

Chugh A, Amin J, Shea MJ. Diagnosis and management of stable coronary artery disease. *Clinics in Family Practice* 2001; 3(4).

Clinical features of angina pectoris. In: Noble J, Greene HL, editors. *Textbook of primary care medicine.* St. Louis: Mosby, 2001.

D'Agostino RB, Russell MW, Huse DM, Ellison RC, Silbershatz H, Wilson PW et al. Primary and subsequent coronary risk appraisal: new results from the Framingham study. *Am Heart J* 2000; 139(2 Pt 1):272–281.

Dankner R, Goldbourt U, Boyko V, Reicher-Reiss H. Predictors of cardiac and noncardiac mortality among 14,697 patients with coronary heart disease. *Am J Cardiol* 2003; 91(2):121–127.

De Smet PA. Herbal remedies. *N Engl J Med* 2002; 347(25):2046–2056.

Eaton CB. Can reduced or modified dietary fat prevent cardiovascular disease? *Am Fam Physician* 2002; 65(1):53–55.

Gavagan T. Cardiovascular disease. *Prim Care* 2002; 29(2):323–38, vi.

Grundy SM. Alternative approaches to cholesterol-lowering therapy. *Am J Cardiol* 2002; 90(10):1135–1138.

Havranek EP. Primary prevention of CHD: nine ways to reduce risk. *Am Fam Physician* 1999; 59(6):1455–1463, 1466.

He J, Whelton PK. Elevated systolic blood pressure and risk of cardiovascular and renal disease: overview of evidence from observational epidemiologic studies and randomized controlled trials. *Am Heart J* 1999; 138(3 Pt 2):211–219.

Heidenreich PA, McClellan M. Trends in treatment and outcomes for acute myocardial infarction: 1975–1995. *Am J Med* 2001; 110(3):165–174.

Hennekens CH. Update on aspirin in the treatment and prevention of cardiovascular disease. *Am Heart J* 1999; 137(4 Pt 2):S9–S13.

Jacobson TA. Clinical context: current concepts of coronary heart disease management. *Am J Med* 2001; 110 (Suppl 6A):3S–11S.

Keevil JG, Stein JH, McBride PE. Cardiovascular disease prevention. *Prim Care* 2002; 29(3):667–696.

Kuritzky L. Atherosclerotic vascular disease: management of angina in the office setting. *Prim Care* 2000; 27(3):615–629, vi.

Mehr DR, Tatum PE, III. Primary prevention of disease of old age. *Clin Geriatr Med* 2002; 18(3):407–430.

Mukamal KJ, Mittleman MA, Maclure M, Sherwood JB, Goldberg RJ, Muller JE. Recent aspirin use is associated with smaller myocardial infarct size and lower likelihood of Q-wave infarction. *Am Heart J* 1999; 137(6): 1120–1128.

Rosengren A. Improved diet and lifestyle in middle-aged women helped reduce the incidence of CHD: a combination of diet, exercise, alcohol consumption, body-mass index and non-smoking status is associated with a very low risk of CHD among women. *Evidence-based Cardiovascular Medicine* 2000; 4(4):92–94.

Stein EA. Identification and treatment of individuals at high risk of coronary heart disease. *Am J Med* 2002; 112 (Suppl 8A):3S–9S.

Torres MR, Short L, Baglin T, Case C, Gibbs H, Marwick TH. Usefulness of clinical risk markers and ischemic threshold to stratify risk in patients undergoing major noncardiac surgery. *Am J Cardiol* 2002; 90(3):238–242.

Ueda K, Takahashi M, Ozawa K, Kinoshita M. Decreased soluble interleukin-6 receptor in patients with acute myocardial infarction. *Am Heart J* 1999; 138(5 Pt 1):908–915.

Zanger DR, Solomon AJ, Gersh BJ. Contemporary management of angina: part I. Risk assessment. *Am Fam Physician* 1999; 60(9):2543–2552.

————. Contemporary management of angina: part II. Medical management of chronic stable angina. *Am Fam Physician* 2000; 61(1):129–138.

HERBALS

Che H, Luo K. Effects of huang qi wu wu decoction on plasma proteins in 70 cases of chronic pulmonary heart disease. *J Tradit Chin Med* 2000; 20(4):254–257.

Chen TH, Liu JC, Chang JJ, Tsai MF, Hsieh MH, Chan P. The in vitro inhibitory effect of flavonoid astilbin on 3-hydroxy-3-methylglutaryl coenzyme A reductase on Vero cells. *Zhonghua Yi Xue Za Zhi* (Taipei) 2001; 64(7): 382–387.

Chopra A. Ayurvedic medicine and arthritis. *Rheum Dis Clin North Am* 2000; 26(1):133–144, x.

De Smet PA. Herbal remedies. *N Engl J Med* 2002; 347(25):2046–2056.

Durrington PN, Bhatnagar D, Mackness MI, Morgan J, Julier K, Khan MA et al. An omega-3 polyunsaturated fatty acid concentrate administered for one year decreased triglycerides in simvastatin treated patients with coronary heart disease and persisting hypertriglyceridaemia. *Heart* 2001; 85(5): 544–548.

Ernst E, Chrubasik S. Phyto-anti-inflammatories. A systematic review of randomized, placebo-controlled, double-blind trials. *Rheum Dis Clin North Am* 2000; 26(1):13–27, vii.

Ernst E, Pittler MH. Herbal medicine. *Med Clin North Am* 2002; 86(1):149–161.

Heber D, Lembertas A, Lu QY, Bowerman S, Go VL. An analysis of nine proprietary Chinese red yeast rice dietary supplements: implications of variability in chemical profile and contents. *J Altern Complement Med* 2001; 7(2):133–139.

Holub BJ. Clinical nutrition: 4. Omega-3 fatty acids in cardiovascular care. *CMAJ* 2002; 166(5):608–615.

Marcus DM, Grollman AP. Botanical medicines—the need for new regulations. *N Engl J Med* 2002; 347(25):2073–2076.

Massey PB. Dietary supplements. *Med Clin North Am* 2002; 86(1):127–147.

Morelli V, Zoorob RJ. Alternative therapies: part II. Congestive heart failure and hypercholesterolemia. *Am Fam Physician* 2000; 62(6):1325–1330.

Panush RS. Preface. *Rheum Dis Clin North Am* 2000; 26(1).

Paul B, Masih I, Deopujari J, Charpentier C. Occurrence of resveratrol and pterostilbene in age-old darakchasava, an ayurvedic medicine from India. *J Ethnopharmacol* 1999; 68(1–3):71–76.

Pearce KA, Boosalis MG, Yeager B. Update on vitamin supplements for the prevention of coronary disease and stroke. *Am Fam Physician* 2000; 62(6):1359–1366.

Qiu R, He J. Effects of xin mai tong capsule on vasoregulatory peptides in the patients of coronary heart disease. *J Tradit Chin Med* 2000; 20(4):251–253.

Roche BSc MPH. Omega-3 fatty acid concentrate decreased triglycerides in coronary heart disease patients treated with simvastatin. *Evidence-based Cardiovascular Medicine* 2001; 5(3):104–105.

Straus SE. Herbal medicines—what's in the bottle? *N Engl J Med* 2002; 347(25):1997–1998.

Tao X, Lipsky PE. The Chinese anti-inflammatory and immunosuppressive herbal remedy Tripterygium wilfordii Hook F. *Rheum Dis Clin North Am* 2000; 26(1):29–50, viii.

Wang N, Minatoguchi S, Uno Y, Arai M, Hashimoto K, Hashimoto Y et al. Treatment with sheng-mai-san reduces myocardial infarct size through activation of protein kinase C and opening of mitochondrial KATP channel. *Am J Chin Med* 2001; 29(2):367–375.

Zhou S, Shao W, Duan C. [Observation of preventing and treating effect of Salvia miltiorrhiza composita on patients with ischemic coronary heart disease undergoing non-heart surgery]. *Zhongguo Zhong Xi Yi Jie He Za Zhi* 1999; 19(2):75–76.

INFECTIOUS DISEASE

Aldous MB, Grayston JT, Wang SP, Foy HM. Seroepidemiology of Chlamydia pneumoniae TWAR infection in Seattle families, 1966–1979. *J Infect Dis* 1992; 166(3):646–649.

Allegra L, Blasi F, Centanni S, Cosentini R, Denti F, Raccanelli R et al. Acute exacerbations of asthma in adults: role of Chlamydia pneumoniae infection. *Eur Respir J* 1994; 7(12):2165–2168.

Augenbraun MH, Roblin PM, Chirgwin K, Landman D, Hammerschlag MR. Isolation of Chlamydia pneumoniae from the lungs of patients infected with the human immunodeficiency virus. *J Clin Microbiol* 1991; 29(2):401–402.

Augenbraun MH, Roblin PM, Mandel LJ, Hammerschlag MR, Schachter J. Chlamydia pneumoniae pneumonia with pleural effusion: diagnosis by culture. *Am J Med* 1991; 91(4):437–438.

Bates JH, Campbell GD, Barron AL, McCracken GA, Morgan PN, Moses EB et al. Microbial etiology of acute pneumonia in hospitalized patients. *Chest* 1992; 101(4):1005–1012.

Blasi F, Cosentini R, Denti F, Allegra L. Two family outbreaks of Chlamydia pneumoniae infection. *Eur Respir J* 1994; 7(1):102–104.

Blasi F, Denti F, Erba M, Cosentini R, Raccanelli R, Rinaldi A et al. Detection of Chlamydia pneumoniae but not Helicobacter pylori in atherosclerotic plaques of aortic aneurysms. *J Clin Microbiol* 1996; 34(11):2766–2769.

Blasi F, Rizzato G, Gambacorta M, Cosentini R, Raccanelli R, Tarsia P et al. Failure to detect the presence of Chlamydia pneumoniae in sarcoid pathology specimens. *Eur Respir J* 1997; 10(11):2609–2611.

Block S, Hedrick J, Hammerschlag MR, Cassell GH, Craft JC. Mycoplasma pneumoniae and Chlamydia pneumoniae in pediatric community-acquired pneumonia: comparative efficacy and safety of clarithromycin vs. erythromycin ethylsuccinate. *Pediatr Infect Dis J* 1995; 14(6):471–477.

Block SL, Hammerschlag MR, Hedrick J, Tyler R, Smith A, Roblin P et al.

Chlamydia pneumoniae in acute otitis media. *Pediatr Infect Dis J* 1997; 16(9):858–862.

Braun J, Laitko S, Treharne J, Eggens U, Wu P, Distler A et al. Chlamydia pneumoniae—a new causative agent of reactive arthritis and undifferentiated oligoarthritis. *Ann Rheum Dis* 1994; 53(2):100–105.

Burian K, Kis Z, Virok D, Endresz V, Prohaszka Z, Duba J et al. Independent and joint effects of antibodies to human heat-shock protein 60 and Chlamydia pneumoniae infection in the development of coronary atherosclerosis. *Circulation* 2001; 103(11):1503–1508.

Caldwell HD, Kromhout J, Schachter J. Purification and partial characterization of the major outer membrane protein of Chlamydia trachomatis. *Infect Immun* 1981; 31(3):1161–1176.

Campbell LA, O'Brien ER, Cappuccio AL, Kuo CC, Wang SP, Stewart D et al. Detection of Chlamydia pneumoniae TWAR in human coronary atherectomy tissues. *J Infect Dis* 1995; 172(2):585–588.

Campbell LA, Perez MM, Hamilton DJ, Kuo CC, Grayston JT. Detection of Chlamydia pneumoniae by polymerase chain reaction. *J Clin Microbiol* 1992; 30(2):434–439.

Castell DO. Do chronic infections play a role in the genesis of atherosclerosis? *Medscape Cardiology* 2001;5(1).

Chandra HR, Choudhary N, O'Neill C, Boura J, Timmis GC, O'Neill WW. Chlamydia pneumoniae exposure and inflammatory markers in acute coronary syndrome (CIMACS). *Am J Cardiol* 2001; 88(3):214–218.

Chirgwin K, Roblin PM, Gelling M, Hammerschlag MR, Schachter J. Infection with Chlamydia pneumoniae in Brooklyn. *J Infect Dis* 1991; 163(4): 757–761.

Chiu B, Viira E, Tucker W, Fong IW. Chlamydia pneumoniae, cytomegalovirus, and herpes simplex virus in atherosclerosis of the carotid artery. *Circulation* 1997; 96(7):2144–2148.

Clark R, Mushatt D, Fazal B. Case report: Chlamydia pneumoniae pneumonia in an HIV-infected man. *Am J Med Sci* 1991; 302(3):155–156.

Comandini UV, Maggi P, Santopadre P, Monno R, Angarano G, Vullo V. Chlamydia pneumoniae respiratory infections among patients infected with the human immunodeficiency virus. *Eur J Clin Microbiol Infect Dis* 1997; 16(10):720–726.

Cook PJ, Honeybourne D, Lip GY, Beevers DG, Wise R, Davies P. Chlamydia pneumoniae antibody titers are significantly associated with acute stroke and transient cerebral ischemia: the West Birmingham Stroke Project. *Stroke* 1998; 29(2):404–410.

Cosentini R, Blasi F, Raccanelli R, Rossi S, Arosio C, Tarsia P et al. Severe community-acquired pneumonia: a possible role for Chlamydia pneumoniae. *Respiration* 1996; 63(2):61–65.

Cox RL, Kuo CC, Grayston JT, Campbell LA. Deoxiribonucleic-acid relatedness of chlamydia sp strain TWAR to clamydia-trachmatis and chlamydia-psittaci. *Internat J System Bacteriol* 1988; 38(3):265–268.

Dalhoff K, Maass M. Chlamydia pneumoniae pneumonia in hospitalized patients. Clinical characteristics and diagnostic value of polymerase chain reaction detection in BAL. *Chest* 1996;110(2):351–356.

Einarsson S, Sigurdsson HK, Magnusdottir SD, Erlendsdottir H, Briem H, Gudmundsson S. Age specific prevalence of antibodies against Chlamydia pneumoniae in Iceland. *Scand J Infect Dis* 1994; 26(4):393–397.

Ekman MR, Grayston JT, Visakorpi R, Kleemola M, Kuo CC, Saikku P. An epidemic of infections due to Chlamydia pneumoniae in military conscripts. *Clin Infect Dis* 1993; 17(3):420–425.

Emre U, Bernius M, Roblin PM, Gaerlan PF, Summersgill JT, Steiner P et al. Chlamydia pneumoniae infection in patients with cystic fibrosis. *Clin Infect Dis* 1996; 22(5):819–823.

Emre U, Roblin PM, Gelling M, Dumornay W, Rao M, Hammerschlag MR et al. The association of Chlamydia pneumoniae infection and reactive airway disease in children. *Arch Pediatr Adolesc Med* 1994; 148(7):727–732.

Emre U, Sokolovskaya N, Roblin PM, Schachter J, Hammerschlag MR. Detection of anti-Chlamydia pneumoniae IgE in children with reactive airway disease. *J Infect Dis* 1995; 172(1):265–267.

Erntell M, Ljunggren K, Gadd T, Persson K. Erythema nodosum—a manifestation of Chlamydia pneumoniae (strain TWAR) infection. *Scand J Infect Dis* 1989; 21(6):693–696.

Fang GD, Fine M, Orloff J, Arisumi D, Yu VL, Kapoor W et al. New and emerging etiologies for community-acquired pneumonia with implications for therapy. A prospective multicenter study of 359 cases. *Medicine* (Baltimore) 1990; 69(5):307–316.

File TM, Jr., Segreti J, Dunbar L, Player R, Kohler R, Williams RR et al. A multicenter, randomized study comparing the efficacy and safety of intravenous and/or oral levofloxacin versus ceftriaxone and/or cefuroxime axetil in treatment of adults with community-acquired pneumonia. *Antimicrob Agents Chemother* 1997; 41(9):1965–1972.

Fong IW, Chiu B, Viira E, Fong MW, Jang D, Mahony J. Rabbit model for Chlamydia pneumoniae infection. *J Clin Microbiol* 1997; 35(1):48–52.

Forgie IM, O'Neill KP, Lloyd-Evans N, Leinonen M, Campbell H, Whittle HC et al. Etiology of acute lower respiratory tract infections in Gambian children: I. Acute lower respiratory tract infections in infants presenting at the hospital. *Pediatr Infect Dis J* 1991; 10(1):33–41.

―――. Etiology of acute lower respiratory tract infections in Gambian children: II. Acute lower respiratory tract infection in children ages one to nine years presenting at the hospital. *Pediatr Infect Dis J* 1991; 10(1): 42–47.

Forsey T, Darougar S, Treharne JD. Prevalence in human beings of antibodies to Chlamydia IOL-207, an atypical strain of chlamydia. *J Infect Dis* 1986; 12(2):145–152.

Foy HM, Kenny GE, Cooney MK, Allan ID. Long-term epidemiology of infections with Mycoplasma pneumoniae. *J Infect Dis* 1979; 139(6):681–687.

Fryden A, Kihlstrom E, Maller R, Persson K, Romanus V, Ansehn S. A clinical and epidemiological study of "ornithosis" caused by Chlamydia psittaci and Chlamydia pneumoniae (strain TWAR). *Scand J Infect Dis* 1989; 21(6):681–691.

Fryer RH, Schwobe EP, Woods ML, Rodgers GM. Chlamydia species infect human vascular endothelial cells and induce procoagulant activity. *J Investig Med* 1997; 45(4):168–174.

Gaydos CA, Eiden JJ, Oldach D, Mundy LM, Auwaerter P, Warner ML et al. Diagnosis of Chlamydia pneumoniae infection in patients with community-acquired pneumonia by polymerase chain reaction enzyme immunoassay. *Clin Infect Dis* 1994; 19(1):157–160.

Gaydos CA, Fowler CL, Gill VJ, Eiden JJ, Quinn TC. Detection of Chlamydia pneumoniae by polymerase chain reaction-enzyme immunoassay in an immunocompromised population. *Clin Infect Dis* 1993; 17(4):718–723.

Gaydos CA, Quinn TC, Eiden JJ. Identification of Chlamydia pneumoniae by DNA amplification of the 16S rRNA gene. *J Clin Microbiol* 1992; 30(4):796–800.

Gaydos CA, Roblin PM, Hammerschlag MR, Hyman CL, Eiden JJ, Schachter J et al. Diagnostic utility of PCR-enzyme immunoassay, culture, and serology for detection of Chlamydia pneumoniae in symptomatic and asymptomatic patients. *J Clin Microbiol* 1994; 32(4):903–905.

Gaydos CA, Summersgill JT, Sahney NN, Ramirez JA, Quinn TC. Replication of Chlamydia pneumoniae in vitro in human macrophages, endothelial cells, and aortic artery smooth muscle cells. *Infect Immun* 1996; 64(5):1614–1620.

Girard SE, Temesgen Z. Emerging concepts in disease management: a role for antimicrobial therapy in coronary artery disease. *Expert Opin Pharmacother* 2001; 2(5):765–772.

Gnarpe J, Gnarpe H, Sundelof B. Endemic prevalence of Chlamydia pneumoniae in subjectively healthy persons. *Scand J Infect Dis* 1991; 23(3):387–388.

Godzik KL, O'Brien ER, Wang SK, Kuo CC. In vitro susceptibility of human vascular wall cells to infection with Chlamydia pneumoniae. *J Clin Microbiol* 1995; 33(9):2411–2414.

Gray GC, McPhate DC, Leinonen M, Cassell GH, Deperalta EP, Putnam SD et al. Weekly oral azithromycin as prophylaxis for agents causing acute respiratory disease. *Clin Infect Dis* 1998; 26(1):103–110.

Grayston JT. Chlamydia pneumoniae (TWAR) infections in children. *Pediatr Infect Dis J* 1994; 13(8):675–684.

Grayston JT. Infections caused by Chlamydia pneumoniae strain TWAR. *Clin Infect Dis* 1992; 15(5):757–761.

Grayston JT, Aldous MB, Easton A, Wang SP, Kuo CC, Campbell LA et al. Evidence that Chlamydia pneumoniae causes pneumonia and bronchitis. *J Infect Dis* 1993; 168(5):1231–1235.

Grayston JT, Diwan VK, Cooney M, Wang SP. Community- and hospital-acquired pneumonia associated with Chlamydia TWAR infection demonstrated serologically. *Arch Intern Med* 1989; 149(1):169–173.

Grayston JT, Kuo CC, Campbell LA, Wang SP. Chlamydia-pneumoniae sp-nov for chlamydia sp strain TWAR. *Internat J System Bacteriol* 1989; 39(1):88–90.

Grayston JT, Kuo CC, Coulson AS, Campbell LA, Lawrence RD, Lee MJ et al. Chlamydia pneumoniae (TWAR) in atherosclerosis of the carotid artery. *Circulation* 1995; 92(12):3397–3400.

Grayston JT, Kuo CC, Wang SP, Altman J. A new Chlamydia psittaci strain, TWAR, isolated in acute respiratory tract infections. *N Engl J Med* 1986; 315(3):161–168.

Grayston JT, Mordhorst C, Bruu AL, Vene S, Wang SP. Countrywide epidemics of Chlamydia pneumoniae, strain TWAR, in Scandinavia, 1981–1983. *J Infect Dis* 1989; 159(6):1111–1114.

Gupta S. Chlamydia pneumoniae, monocyte activation, and azithromycin in coronary heart disease. *Am Heart J* 1999; 138(5 Pt 2):S539–S541.

Gupta S, Leatham EW, Carrington D, Mendall MA, Kaski JC, Camm AJ. Elevated Chlamydia pneumoniae antibodies, cardiovascular events, and azithromycin in male survivors of myocardial infarction. *Circulation* 1997; 96(2):404–407.

Gurfinkel E, Bozovich G, Daroca A, Beck E, Mautner B. Randomised trial of roxithromycin in non-Q-wave coronary syndromes: ROXIS pilot study. *Lancet* 1997; 350(9075):404–407.

Hahn DL, Anttila T, Saikku P. Association of Chlamydia pneumoniae IgA antibodies with recently symptomatic asthma. *Epidemiol Infect* 1996; 117(3):513–517.

Hahn DL, Dodge RW, Golubjatnikov R. Association of Chlamydia pneumoniae (strain TWAR) infection with wheezing, asthmatic bronchitis, and adult-onset asthma. *JAMA* 1991; 266(2):225–230.

Hahn DL, Golubjatnikov R. Asthma and chlamydial infection: a case series. *J Fam Pract* 1994; 38(6):589–595.

Haidl S, Ivarsson S, Bjerre I, Persson K. Guillain-Barre-Syndrome after chlamydia-pneumoniae infection. *N Engl J Med* 1992; 326(8):576–577.

Haidl S, Sveger T, Persson K. Longitudinal pattern of antibodies to Chlamydia pneumoniae in children. In: Orfila J, Byrne GI, Chernesky MA et al., editors. *Chlamydia infections*. Bologna: Societa Editrice Esculapio, 1994.

Hammerschlag MR. Chirgwin K. Roblin PM, Gelling M, Dumornay W, Mandel L et al. Persistent infection with Chlamydia pneumoniae following acute respiratory illness. *Clin Infect Dis* 1992; 14(1):178–182.

Hammerschlag MR, Hyman CL, Roblin PM. In vitro activities of five quinolones against Chlamydia pneumoniae. *Antimicrob Agents Chemother* 1992; 36(3):682–683.

Hammerschlag MR, Qumei KK, Roblin PM. In vitro activities of azithromycin, clarithromycin, L-ofloxacin, and other antibiotics against chlamydia-pneumoniae. *Antimicrob Agents Chemother* 1992; 36(7):1573–1574.

Hyman CL, Augenbraun MH, Roblin PM, Schachter J, Hammerschlag MR. Asymptomatic respiratory-tract infection with chlamydia-pneumoniae TWAR. *J Clin Microbiol* 1991; 29(9):2082–2083.

Hyman CL, Roblin PM, Gaydos CA, Quinn TC, Schachter J, Hammerschlag MR. Prevalence of asymptomatic nasopharyngeal carriage of Chlamydia pneumoniae in subjectively healthy adults: assessment by polymerase chain reaction-enzyme immunoassay and culture. *Clin Infect Dis* 1995; 20(5):1174–1178.

Jackson LA, Campbell LA, Kuo CC, Rodriguez DI, Lee A, Grayston JT. Isolation of Chlamydia pneumoniae from a carotid endarterectomy specimen. *J Infect Dis* 1997; 176(1):292–295.

Jackson LA, Campbell LA, Schmidt RA, Kuo CC, Cappuccio AL, Lee MJ et al. Specificity of detection of Chlamydia pneumoniae in cardiovascular atheroma: evaluation of the innocent bystander hypothesis. *Am J Pathol* 1997; 150(5):1785–1790.

Jackson LA, Grayston JT. Chlamydia pneumoniae. In: Mandell GL, Bennett JE, Dolin R, editors. *Mandell, Douglas, and Bennett's principles and practice of infectious diseases.* Philadelphia: Churchill Livingston, 2000; 2007–2014.

Jantos CA, Wienpahl B, Schiefer HG, Wagner F, Hegemann JH. Infection with Chlamydia pneumoniae in infants and children with acute lower respiratory tract disease. *Pediatr Infect Dis J* 1995; 14(2):117–122.

Jones RB, Batteiger BE. Introduction to chlamydial diseases. In: Mandell GL, Douglas RG, Bennett JE, Dolin R, editors. *Mandell, Douglas, and Bennett's principles and practice of infectious diseases.* Philadelphia: Churchill Livingstone, 2000.

Juvonen J, Juvonen T, Laurila A, Alakarppa H, Lounatmaa K, Surcel HM et al. Demonstration of Chlamydia pneumoniae in the walls of abdominal aortic aneurysms. *J Vasc Surg* 1997; 25(3):499–505.

Kalayoglu MV, Byrne GI. Induction of macrophage foam cell formation by Chlamydia pneumoniae. *J Infect Dis* 1998; 177(3):725–729.

Kaltenboeck B, Kousoulas KG, Storz J. Structures of and allelic diversity and relationships among the major outer membrane protein (ompA) genes of the four chlamydial species. *J Bacteriol* 1993; 175(2):487–502.

Kanamoto Y, Ouchi K, Mizui M, Ushio M, Usui T. Prevalence of antibody to Chlamydia pneumoniae TWAR in Japan. *J Clin Microbiol* 1991; 29(4):816–818.

Karvonen M, Tuomilehto J, Naukkarinen A, Saikku P. The prevalence and regional distribution of antibodies against Chlamydia pneumoniae (strain TWAR) in Finland in 1958. *Int J Epidemiol* 1992; 21(2):391–398.

Karvonen M, Tuomilehto J, Pitkaniemi J, Naukkarinen A, Saikku P. Importance of smoking for Chlamydia pneumoniae seropositivity. *Int J Epidemiol* 1994; 23(6):1315–1321.

Kauppinen MT, Lahde S, Syrjala H. Roentgenographic findings of pneumonia caused by Chlamydia pneumoniae. A comparison with streptococcus pneumonia. *Arch Intern Med* 1996; 156(16):1851–1856.

Kauppinen MT, Saikku P, Kujala P, Herva E, Syrjala H. Clinical picture of community-acquired Chlamydia pneumoniae pneumonia requiring hospital treatment: a comparison between chlamydial and pneumococcal pneumonia. *Thorax* 1996; 51(2):185–189.

Kese D, Hren-Vencelj H, Socan M, Beovic B, Cizman M. Prevalence of antibodies to Chlamydia pneumoniae in Slovenia. *Eur J Clin Microbiol Infect Dis* 1994; 13(6):523–525.

Kishimoto T, Kimura M, Kubota Y, et al. An outbreak of C. pneumoniae infection in households and schools. In: Orfila J, Byrne GI, Chernesky MA et al., editors. *Chlamydial infections.* Bologna: Societa Editrice Esculapio, 1994; 465–468.

Kleemola M, Saikku P, Visakorpi R, Wang SP, Grayston JT. Epidemics of pneumonia caused by TWAR, a new Chlamydia organism, in military trainees in Finland. J *Infect Dis* 1988; 157(2):230–236.

Knoebel E, Vijayagopal P, Figueroa JE, Martin DH. In vitro infection of smooth muscle cells by Chlamydia pneumoniae. *Infect Immun* 1997; 65 (2):503–506.

Koskiniemi M, Gencay M, Salonen O, Puolakkainen M, Farkkila M, Saikku P et al. Chlamydia pneumoniae associated with central nervous system infections. *Eur Neurol* 1996; 36(3):160–163.

Koskiniemi M, Korppi M, Mustonen K, Rantala H, Muttilainen M, Herrgard E et al. Epidemiology of encephalitis in children. A prospective multicentre study. *Eur J Pediatr* 1997; 156(7):541–545.

Kuo CC, Chen HH, Wang SP, Grayston JT, Identification of a new group of Chlamydia psittaci strains called TWAR. *J Clin Microbiol* 1986; 24(6):1034–1037.

Kuo CC, Coulson AS, Campbell LA, Cappuccio AL, Lawrence RD, Wang SP et al. Detection of Chlamydia pneumoniae in atherosclerotic plaques in the walls of arteries of lower extremities from patients undergoing bypass operation for arterial obstruction. *J Vasc Surg* 1997; 26(1):29–31.

Kuo CC, Chi EY, Grayston JT. Ultrastructural study of entry of Chlamydia strain TWAR into HeLa cells. *Infect Immun* 1988; 56(6):1668–1672.

Kuo CC, Gown AM, Benditt EP, Grayston JT. Detection of Chlamydia pneumoniae in aortic lesions of atherosclerosis by immunocytochemical stain. *Arterioscler Thromb* 1993; 13(10):1501–1504.

Kuo CC, Grayston JT. Factors affecting viability and growth in HeLa 229 cells of Chlamydia sp. strain TWAR. *J Clin Microbiol* 1988; 26(5):812–815.

Kuo CC, Grayston JT. In vitro drug susceptibility of Chlamydia sp. strain TWAR. *Antimicrob Agents Chemother* 1988; 32(2):257–258.

Kuo CC, Grayston JT. A sensitive cell line, HL cells, for isolation and propagation of Chlamydia pneumoniae strain TWAR. *J Infect Dis* 1990; 162(3):755–758.

Kuo CC, Grayston JT, Campbell LA, Goo YA, Wissler RW, Benditt EP. Chlamydia pneumoniae (TWAR) in coronary arteries of young adults (15–34 years old). *Proc Natl Acad Sci USA* 1995; 92(15):6911–6914.

Kuo CC, Jackson LA, Lee A, Grayston JT. In vitro activities of azithromycin, clarithromycin, and other antibiotics against Chlamydia pneumoniae. *Antimicrob Agents Chemother* 1996; 40(11):2669–2670.

Kuo CC, Shor A, Campbell LA, Fukushi H, Patton DL, Grayston JT. Demonstration of Chlamydia pneumoniae in atherosclerotic lesions of coronary arteries. *J Infect Dis* 1993; 167(4):841–849.

Kuvin JT, Kimmelstiel CD. Infectious causes of atherosclerosis. *Am Heart J* 1999; 137(2):216–226.

Laitinen K, Laurila A, Pyhala L, Leinonen M, Saikku P. Chlamydia pneumoniae infection induces inflammatory changes in the aortas of rabbits. *Infect Immun* 1997; 65(11):4832–4835.

Laurila AL, Anttila T, Laara E, Bloigu A, Virtamo J, Albanes D et al. Serological evidence of an association between Chlamydia pneumoniae infection and lung cancer. *Int J Cancer* 1997; 74(1):31–34.

Linnanmaki E, Leinonen M, Mattila K, Nieminen MS, Valtonen V, Saikku P. Chlamydia pneumoniae–specific circulating immune complexes in patients with chronic coronary heart disease. *Circulation* 1993; 87(4): 1130–1134.

Maass M, Bartels C, Engel PM, Mamat U, Sievers HH. Endovascular presence of viable Chlamydia pneumoniae is a common phenomenon in coronary artery disease. *J Am Coll Cardiol* 1998; 31(4):827–832.

Marrie TJ, Durant H, Yates L. Community-acquired pneumonia requiring hospitalization: 5-year prospective study. *Rev Infect Dis* 1989; 11(4):586–599.

Marrie TJ, Grayston JT, Wang SP, Kuo CC. Pneumonia associated with the TWAR strain of Chlamydia. *Ann Intern Med* 1987; 106(4):507–511.

Marrie TJ, Harczy M, Mann OE, Landymore RW, Raza A, Wang SP et al. Culture-negative endocarditis probably due to Chlamydia pneumoniae. *J Infect Dis* 1990; 161(1):127–129.

Marston BJ, Plouffe JF, File TM, Jr., Hackman BA, Salstrom SJ, Lipman HB et al. Incidence of community-acquired pneumonia requiring hospitalization. Results of a population-based active surveillance Study in Ohio. The Community-Based Pneumonia Incidence Study Group. *Arch Intern Med* 1997; 157(15): 1709–1718.

Marton A, Karolyi A, Szalka A. Prevalence of Chlamydia pneumoniae antibodies in Hungary. *Eur J Clin Microbiol Infect Dis* 1992; 11(2):139–142.

McConnell CT, Jr., Plouffe JF, File TM, Mueller CF, Wong KH, Skelton SK et al. Radiographic appearance of Chlamydia pneumoniae (TWAR strain) respiratory infections. CBPIS Study Group. Community-based Pneumonia Incidence Study. *Radiology* 1994; 192(3):819–824.

Melgosa MP, Kuo CC, Campbell LA. Outer membrane complex proteins of Chlamydia pneumoniae. *FEMS Microbiol Lett* 1993; 112(2):199–204.

Melnick SL, Shahar E, Folsom AR, Grayston JT, Sorlie PD, Wang SP et al. Past infection by Chlamydia pneumoniae strain TWAR and asymptomatic carotid atherosclerosis. Atherosclerosis Risk in Communities (ARIC) Study Investigators. *Am J Med* 1993; 95(5):499–504.

Mendall MA, Carrington D, Strachan D, Patel P, Molineaux N, Levi J et al. Chlamydia pneumoniae: risk factors for seropositivity and association with coronary heart disease. *J Infect* 1995; 30(2):121–128.

Michel D, Antoine JC, Pozzetto B, Gaudin OG, Lucht F. Lumbosacral meningoradiculitis associated with Chlamydia pneumoniae infection. *J Neurol Neurosurg Psychiatry* 1992; 55(6):511.

Miller ST, Hammerschlag MR, Chirgwin K, Rao SP, Roblin P, Gelling M et al. Role of Chlamydia pneumoniae in acute chest syndrome of sickle cell disease. *J Pediatr* 1991; 118(1):30–33.

Miyashita N, Niki Y, Nakajima M, Fukano H, Matsushima T. Prevalence of asymptomatic infection with Chlamydia pneumoniae in subjectively health adults. *Chest* 2001; 119(5):1416–1419.

Moazed TC, Campbell LA, Rosenfeld ME. Chlamydia pneumoniae infection accelerates the progression of atherosclerosis in apolipoprotein (Apo-E)-deficient mice. In: Stephens RS, Byrne GI, Clarke IN, Christiansen G, editors. *Chlamydial infections: proceedings of the Ninth International Symposium on Human Chlamydial Infection.* San Francisco: International Chlamydia Symposium, 1998; 426–429.

Moazed TC, Kuo C, Grayston JT, Campbell LA. Murine models of Chlamydia pneumoniae infection and atherosclerosis. *J Infect Dis* 1997; 175(4): 883–890.

Montes M, Cilla G, Alcorta M, Perez-Trallero E. High prevalence of Chlamydia pneumoniae infection in children and young adults in Spain. *Pediatr Infect Dis J* 1992; 11(11):972–973.

Mordhorst CH, Wang AP, Grayston JT. Transmission of C. pneumoniae (TWAR). In: Orfila J, Byrne GI, Chernesky MA et al., editors. *Chlamydial Infections.* Bologna: Societa Editrice Esculapio, 1994; 488–491.

Mordhorst CH, Wang SP, Grayston JT. Outbreak of Chlamydia pneumoniae infection in four farm families. *Eur J Clin Microbiol Infect Dis* 1992; 11(7):617–620.

Muhlestein JB, Anderson JL, Hammond EH, Zhao L, Trehan S, Schwobe EP et al. Infection with Chlamydia pneumoniae accelerates the development of atherosclerosis and treatment with azithromycin prevents it in a rabbit model. *Circulation* 1998; 97(7):633–636.

Muhlestein JB, Hammond EH, Carlquist JF, Radicke E, Thomson MJ, Karagounis LA et al. Increased incidence of Chlamydia species within the coronary arteries of patients with symptomatic atherosclerotic versus other forms of cardiovascular disease. *J Am Coll Cardiol* 1996; 27(7):1555–1561.

Myhra W, Mordhorst CH, Wang SP, Grayston JT. Clinical features of Chlamydia pneumoniae, strain TWAR, infection in Denmark 1975–1987. In: Bowie WR, Caldwell HD, Jones RB et al., editors. *Chlamydial infections*. Cambridge: Cambridge University Press, 1990; 422–425.

Ni AP, Lin GY, Yang L, He HY, Huang CW, Liu ZJ et al. A seroepidemiologic study of Chlamydia pneumoniae, Chlamydia trachomatis and Chlamydia psittaci in different populations on the mainland of China. *Scand J Infect Dis* 1996; 28(6):553–557.

Norton R, Schepetiuk S, Kok TW. Chlamydia pneumoniae pneumonia with endocarditis. *Lancet* 1995; 345(8961):1376–1377.

Ogawa H, Fujisawa T, Kazuyama Y. Isolation of Chlamydia pneumoniae from middle ear aspirates of otitis media with effusion: a case report. *J Infect Dis* 1990; 162(4):1000–1001.

Ogawa H, Hashiguchi K, Kazuyama Y. Recovery of Chlamydia pneumoniae, in six patients with otitis media with effusion. *J Laryngol Otol* 1992; 106(6):490–492.

Orr PH, Peeling RW, Fast M, Brunka J, Duckworth H, Harding GK et al. Serological study of responses to selected pathogens causing respiratory tract infection in the institutionalized elderly. *Clin Infect Dis* 1996; 23(6):1240–1245.

Paltiel O, Kark JD, Leinonen M, Saikku P. High prevalence of antibodies to Chlamydia pneumoniae; determinants of IgG and IgA seropositivity among Jerusalem residents. *Epidemiol Infect* 1995; 114(3):465–473.

Patel P, Mendall MA, Carrington D, Strachan DP, Leatham E, Molineaux N et al. Association of Helicobacter pylori and Chlamydia pneumoniae infections with coronary heart disease and cardiovascular risk factors. *BMJ* 1995; 311(7007):711–714.

Patnode D, Wang SP, Grayston JT. Persistence of Chlamydia pneumoniae, strain TWAR, microimmunofluorescent antibody. In: Bowie WR, Caldwell HD, Jones RB et al., editors. *Chlamydial infections*. Cambridge: Cambridge University Press, 1990; 406–409.

Pether JV, Wang SP, Grayston JT. Chlamydia pneumoniae, strain TWAR, as the cause of an outbreak in a boys' school previously called psittacosis. *Epidemiol Infect* 1989; 103(2):395–400.

Porath A, Schlaeffer F, Lieberman D. The epidemiology of community-acquired pneumonia among hospitalized adults. *J Infect* 1997; 34(1):41–48.

Puolakkainen M, Campbell LA, Kuo CC, Leinonen M, Gronhagen-Riska C, Saikku P. Serological response to Chlamydia pneumoniae in patients with sarcoidosis. *J Infect* 1996; 33(3):199–205.

Ramirez JA. Isolation of Chlamydia pneumoniae from the coronary artery of a patient with coronary atherosclerosis. The Chlamydia pneumoniae/Atherosclerosis Study Group. *Ann Intern Med* 1996; 125(12):979–982.

Ramirez JA, Ahkee S, Tolentino A, Miller RD, Summersgill JT. Diagnosis of Legionella pneumophila, Mycoplasma pneumoniae, or Chlamydia pneumoniae lower respiratory infection using the polymerase chain reaction on a single throat swab specimen. *Diagn Microbiol Infect Dis* 1996; 24(1): 7–14.

Saikku P, Leinonen M, Mattila K, Ekman MR, Nieminen MS, Makela PH et al. Serological evidence of an association of a novel Chlamydia, TWAR, with chronic coronary heart disease and acute myocardial infarction. *Lancet* 1988; 2(8618):983–986.

Saikku P, Leinonen M, Tenkanen L, Linnanmaki E, Ekman MR, Manninen V et al. Chronic Chlamydia pneumoniae infection as a risk factor for coronary heart disease in the Helsinki Heart Study. *Ann Intern Med* 1992; 116(4):273–278.

Saikku P, Ruutu P, Leinonen M, Panelius J, Tupasi TE, Grayston JT. Acute lower-respiratory-tract infection associated with chlamydial TWAR antibody in Filipino children. *J Infect Dis* 1988; 158(5):1095–1097.

Saikku P, Wang SP, Kleemola M, Brander E, Rusanen E, Grayston JT. An epidemic of mild pneumonia due to an unusual strain of Chlamydia psittaci. *J Infect Dis* 1985; 151(5):832–839.

Sessa R, Di Pietro M, Santino I, del Piano M, Varveri A, Dagianti A et al. Chlamydia pneumoniae infection and atherosclerotic coronary disease. *Am Heart J* 1999; 137(6): 1116–1119.

Shah PK. Plaque disruption and thrombosis. Potential role of inflammation and infection. *Cardiol Clin* 1999; 17(2):271–281.

Shor A, Kuo CC, Patton DL. Detection of Chlamydia pneumoniae in coronary arterial fatty streaks and atheromatous plaques. *S Afr Med J* 1992; 82(3):158–161.

Steinhoff D, Lode H, Ruckdeschel G, Heidrich B, Rolfs A, Fehrenbach FJ et al. Chlamydia pneumoniae as a cause of community-acquired pneumonia in hospitalized patients in Berlin. *Clin Infect Dis* 1996; 22(6):958–964.

Storgaard M, Ostergaard L, Jensen JS, Farholt S, Larsen K, Ovesen T et al. Chlamydia pneumoniae in children with otitis media. *Clin Infect Dis* 1997; 25(5):1090–1093.

Sundelof B, Gnarpe H, Gnarpe J. An unusual manifestation of Chlamydia pneumoniae infection: meningitis, hepatitis, iritis and atypical erythema nodosum. *Scand J Infect Dis* 1993; 25(2):259–261.

Thom DH, Grayston JT, Campbell LA, Kuo CC, Diwan VK, Wang SP. Respiratory infection with Chlamydia pneumoniae in middle-aged and older adult outpatients. *Eur J Clin Microbiol Infect Dis* 1994; 13(10):785–792.

Thom DH, Grayston JT, Siscovick DS, Wang SP, Weiss NS, Daling JR. Association of prior infection with Chlamydia pneumoniae and angiographically demonstrated coronary artery disease. *JAMA* 1992; 268(1):68–72.

Thom DH, Grayston JT, Wang SP, Kuo CC, Altman J. Chlamydia pneumoniae strain TWAR, Mycoplasma pneumoniae, and viral infections in acute respiratory disease in a university student health clinic population. *Am J Epidemiol* 1990; 132(2):248–256.

Thom DH, Wang SP, Grayston JT, Siscovick DS, Stewart DK, Kronmal RA et al. Chlamydia pneumoniae strain TWAR antibody and angiographically demonstrated coronary artery disease. *Arterioscler Thromb* 1991; 11(3):547–551.

Tong CY, Sillis M. Detection of Chlamydia pneumoniae and Chlamydia psittaci in sputum samples by PCR. *J Clin Pathol* 1993; 46(4):313–317.

Troy CJ, Peeling RW, Ellis AG, Hockin JC, Bennett DA, Murphy MR et al. Chlamydia pneumoniae as a new source of infectious outbreaks in nursing homes. *JAMA* 1997; 277(15):1214–1218.

Valtonen VV. Role of infections in atherosclerosis. *Am Heart J* 1999; 138(5 Pt 2):S431–S433.

Verkooyen RP, Hazenberg MA, Van Haaren GH, Van Den Bosch JM, Snijder RJ, Van Helden HP et al. Age-related interference with Chlamydia pneumoniae microimmunofluorescence serology due to circulating rheumatoid factor. *J Clin Microbiol* 1992; 30(5):1287–1290.

Wang SP, Grayston JT. Microimmunofluorescence serological studies with the TWAR organism. In: Oriel JD, editor. *Chlamydial infections: proceedings of the Sixth International Symposium on Human Chlamydial Infections, Sanderstead, Surrey, 15–21 June 1986.* Cambridge: Cambridge University Press, 1986; 329–332.

Wang SP, Grayston JT. Population prevalence antibody to Chlamydia pneumoniae, strain TWAR. In: Bowie WR, Caldwell HD, Jones RB et al., editors. *Chlamydial infections.* Cambridge: Cambridge University Press, 1990; 402–405.

Wimmer ML, Sandmann-Strupp R, Saikku P, Haberl RL. Association of chlamydial infection with cerebrovascular disease. *Stroke* 1996; 27(12): 2207–2210.

Wright SW, Edwards KM, Decker MD, Grayston JT, Wang S. Prevalence of positive serology for acute Chlamydia pneumoniae infection in emergency department patients with persistent cough. *Acad Emerg Med* 1997; 4(3): 179–183.

Yamashita K, Ouchi K, Shirai M, Gondo T, Nakazawa T, Ito H. Distribution of Chlamydia pneumoniae infection in the athersclerotic carotid artery. *Stroke* 1998; 29(4):773–778.

Yeung SM, McLeod K, Wang SP, Grayston JT, Wang EE. Lack of evidence of Chlamydia pneumoniae infection in infants with acute lower respiratory tract disease. *Eur J Clin Microbiol Infect Dis* 1993; 12(11):850–853.

PUBLIC HEALTH

Berg AO, Atkins D. U.S. Preventive Services Task Force: screening for lipid disorders in adults: recommendations and rationale. *Am J Nurs* 2002; 102(6):91, 93, 95.

Jackson JD. Economics and cost-effectiveness in evaluating the value of cardiovascular therapies. Economics and cost-effectiveness in evaluating the value of cardiovascular therapy: lipid-lowering therapies—an industry perspective. *Am Heart J* 1999; 137(5):S105–S110.

O'Connor GT, O'Connor MA, Beggs V, Nugent WC. What are my chances? *Evidence-based Cardiovascular Medicine* 1999; 3(3):57–58.

Ozminkowski RJ, Goetzel RZ, Smith MW, Cantor RI, Shaughnessy A, Harrison M. The impact of the Citibank, NA, health management program on changes in employee health risks over time. *J Occup Environ Med* 2000; 42(5):502–511.

Pegus C, Bazzarre TL, Brown JS, Menzin J. Effect of the Heart At Work program on awareness of risk factors, self-efficacy, and health behaviors. *J Occup Environ Med* 2002; 44(3):228–236.

Robins SJ. Targeting low high-density lipoprotein cholesterol for therapy: lessons from the Veterans Affairs High-density Lipoprotein Intervention Trial. *Am J Cardiol* 2001; 88(12A):19N–23N.

Safeer RS, Ugalat PS. Cholesterol treatment guidelines update. *Am Fam Physician* 2002; 65(5):871–880.

The National Heart Lung and Blood Institute. Executive summary of the third report of the national cholesterol education program. National Institutes of Health, 2001.

Wasserman J, Whitmer RW, Bazzarre TL, Kennedy ST, Merrick N, Goetzel RZ et al. Gender-specific effects of modifiable health risk factors on coronary heart disease and related expenditures. HERO Research Committee. Health Enhancement Research Organization. *J Occup Environ Med* 2000; 42(11):1060–1069.

STATINS

Ament PW, Bertolino JG, Liszewski JL. Clinically significant drug interactions. *Am Fam Physician* 2000; 61(6):1745–1754.

Amoroso G, Van Boven AJ, Crijns HJ. Drug therapy or coronary angioplasty for the treatment of coronary artery disease: new insights. *Am Heart J* 2001; 141(2 Suppl):S22–S25.

Ansell BJ. Developing a clinical strategy for cholesterol management in an era of unanswered questions. *Am J Cardiol* 2001; 88(4 Suppl):25F–30F.

Azar RR, Waters DD. PRINCE's prospects: statins, inflammation, and coronary risk. *Am Heart J* 2001; 141(6):881–883.

Blair SN, Capuzzi DM, Gottlieb SO, Nguyen T, Morgan JM, Cater NB. Incremental reduction of serum total cholesterol and low-density lipoprotein cholesterol with the addition of plant stanol ester-containing spread to statin therapy. *Am J Cardiol* 2000; 86(1):46–52.

Blumenthal RS. Statins: effective antiatherosclerotic therapy. *Am Heart J* 2000; 139(4):577–583.

Boger RH. Drug interactions of the statins and consequences for drug selection. *Int J Clin Pharmacol Ther* 2001; 39(9):369–382.

Chong PH, Seeger JD, Franklin C. Clinically relevant differences between the statins: implications for therapeutic selection. *Am J Med* 2001; 111(5): 390–400.

Clark LT. Treating dyslipidemia with statins: the risk-benefit profile. *Am Heart J* 2003; 145(3):387–396.

Crouch MA. Effective use of statins to prevent coronary heart disease. *Am Fam Physician* 2001; 63(2):309–304.

Davidson MH. A look to the future: new treatment guidelines and a perspective on statins. *Am J Med* 2002; 112 (Suppl 8A):34S–41S.

Downs JR, Clearfield M, Tyroler HA, Whitney EJ, Kruyer W, Langendorfer A et al. Air Force/Texas Coronary Atherosclerosis Prevention Study (AFCAPS/TEXCAPS): additional perspectives on tolerability of long-term treatment with lovastatin. *Am J Cardiol* 2001; 87(9): 1074–1079.

Dujovne CA. Side effects of statins: hepatitis versus "transaminitis"-myositis versus "CPKitis." *Am J Cardiol* 2002; 89(12):1411–1413.

Gottlieb S. FDA says statin cannot be sold over the counter. *BMJ* 2000; 321(7255):196.

Grundy SM. Alternative approaches to cholesterol-lowering therapy. *Am J Cardiol* 2002; 90(10):1135–1138.

Grundy SM. United States Cholesterol Guidelines 2001: expanded scope of intensive low-density lipoprotein-lowering therapy. *Am J Cardiol* 2001; 88(7B):23J–27J.

Harvard University Gazette. Alpert awards $100,000 for cholesterol research. Harvard University Archives 2000 June 1.

Havranek EP. Primary prevention of CHD: nine ways to reduce risk. *Am Fam Physician* 1999; 59(6):1455–63, 1466.

Hunninghake D, Insull W, Knopp R, Davidson M, Lohrbauer L, Jones P et al. Comparison of the efficacy of atorvastatin versus cerivastatin in primary hypercholesterolemia. *Am J Cardiol* 2001; 88(6):635–639.

Karalis DG, Ross AM, Vacari RM, Zarren H, Scott R. Comparison of efficacy and safety of atorvastatin and simvastatin in patients with dyslipidemia with and without coronary heart disease. *Am J Cardiol* 2002; 89(6):667–671.

Kolata G. U.S. panel backs broader steps to reduce risk of heart attacks. *New York Times* 2001 May 16; A1.

Kreisberg RA, Oberman A. Clinical review 141: lipids and atherosclerosis: lessons learned from randomized controlled trials of lipid lowering and other relevant studies. *J Clin Endocrinol Metab* 2002; 87(2):423–437.

Kwak B, Mulhaupt F, Myit S, Mach F. Statins as a newly recognized type of immunomodulator. *Nat Med* 2000; 6(12):1399–1402.

LaRosa JC. Pleiotropic effects of statins and their clinical significance. *Am J Cardiol* 2001; 88(3):291–293.

LaRosa JC. What do the statins tell us? *Am Heart J* 2002; 144(6 Suppl):S21–S26.

Law MR, Wald NJ, Morris JK, Jordan RE. Value of low dose combination treatment with blood pressure lowering drugs: analysis of 354 randomised trials. *BMJ* 2003; 326(7404):1427.

Law MR, Wald NJ, Rudnicka AR. Quantifying effect of statins on low density lipoprotein cholesterol, ischaemic heart disease, and stroke: systematic review and meta-analysis. *BMJ* 2003; 326(7404):1423.

Nash DT. Need for a moratorium on percutaneous transluminal coronary angioplasty in stable coronary artery disease. *Am J Cardiol* 2002; 89(5): 567–570.

Ong HT. Protecting the heart: a practical review of the statin studies. *MedGenMed* 2002; 4(4):1.

Ornish D. Statins and the soul of medicine. *Am J Cardiol* 2002; 89(11):1286–1290.

Palinski W, Tsimikas S. Immunomodulatory effects of statins: mechanisms and potential impact on arteriosclerosis. *J Am Soc Nephrol* 2002; 13(6): 1673–1681.

Pitt B, Waters D, Brown WV, Van Boven AJ, Schwartz L, Title LM et al. Aggressive lipid-lowering therapy compared with angioplasty in stable coronary artery disease. Atorvastatin versus revascularization treatment investigators. *N Engl J Med* 1999; 341(2):70–76.

Randomised trial of cholesterol lowering in 4444 patients with coronary heart disease: the Scandinavian Simvastatin Survival Study (4S). *Lancet* 1994; 344(8934):1383–1389.

Roberts WC. Getting more people on statins. *Am J Cardiol* 2002; 90(6): 683–685.

Rodgers A. A cure for cardiovascular disease? Combination treatment has enormous potential, especially in developing countries. *BMJ* 2003; 326 (7404):1407–1408.

Rosenson RS. The rationale for combination therapy. *Am J Cardiol* 2002; 90(10B):2K–7K.

Sacks FM. Adherence to statin therapy: why aren't we doing better? *Am J Med* 2002; 113(8):685–686.

Sauvage Nolting PR, Buirma RJ, Hutten BA, Kastelein JJ. Two-year efficacy and safety of simvastatin 80 mg in familial hypercholesterolemia (the Examination of Probands and Relatives in Statin Studies With Familial Hypercholesterolemia [ExPRESS FH]). *Am J Cardiol* 2002; 90(2):181–184.

Schwartz JS. Economics and cost-effectiveness in evaluating the value of cardiovascular therapies. Comparative economic data regarding lipid-lowering drugs. *Am Heart J* 1999; 137(5):S97–104.

Shaywitz DA, Ausiello DA. Discovery: what does the unfolding nature of the statins tell us about the nature of medical breakthroughs? *Harvard Medical Alumni Bulletin* 2001.

Thuraisingham S, Tan KH, Chong KS, Yap SF, Pasamanikam K. A randomised comparison of simvastatin versus simvastatin and low cholesterol diet in the treatment of hypercholesterolaemia. *Int J Clin Pract* 2000; 54(2):78–84.

Tolman KG. The liver and lovastatin. *Am J Cardiol* 2002; 89(12):1374–1380.

Vu D, Murty M, McMorran M. Statins: rhabdomyolysis and myopathy. *CMAJ* 2002; 166(1):85–81.

Wald NJ, Law MR. A strategy to reduce cardiovascular disease by more than 80%. *BMJ* 2003; 326(7404):1419.

Waters DD. Are we aggressive enough in lowering cholesterol? *Am J Cardiol* 2001; 88(4 Suppl): 10F–15F.

Wutz BJ. Hyperlipoproteinemia, Primary (PTG). In: Ferri FF, editor. *Ferri's clinical advisor: instant diagnosis and treatment*. St. Louis: Mosby, 2000.

TESTING

Al Khalili F, Svane B, Wamala SP, Orth-Gomer K, Ryden L, Schenck-Gustafsson K. Clinical importance of risk factors and exercise testing for prediction of significant coronary artery stenosis in women recovering from unstable coronary artery disease: the Stockholm Female Coronary Risk Study. *Am Heart J* 2000; 139(6):971–978.

Alexopoulos D, Toulgaridis T, Davlouros P, Christodoulou J, Sitafidis G, Hahalis G et al. Prognostic significance of coronary artery calcium in asymptomatic subjects with usual cardiovascular risk. *Am Heart J* 2003; 145(3):542–548.

Chugh A, Amin J, Shea MJ. Diagnosis and management of stable coronary artery disease. *Clinics in Family Practice* 2001; 3(4).

Diagnostic Tests. In: Noble J, editor. *Textbook of primary care medicine.* St. Louis: Mosby, 2001.

Henley E. Understanding the risks of medical interventions. *Fam Pract Manag* 2000; 7(5):59–60.

Kiechl S, Egger G, Mayr M, Wiedermann CJ, Bonora E, Oberhollenzer F et al. Chronic infections and the risk of carotid atherosclerosis: prospective results from a large population study. *Circulation* 2001; 103(8):1064–1070.

Meece TL. Stress testing. In: Pfenninger JL, Fowler GC, editors. *Procedures for primary care physicians.* St. Louis: Mosby, 1994.

Myers J, Goebbels U, Dzeikan G, Froelicher V, Bremerich J, Mueller P et al. Exercise training and myocardial remodeling in patients with reduced ventricular function: one-year follow-up with magnetic resonance imaging. *Am Heart J* 2000; 139(2 Pt 1):252–261.

Negrusz-Kawecka M, Kobusiak-Prokopowicz M, Sobotkiewicz-Cyran S, Cyran K. [Incidence of myocardial ischemia in patients with ischemic heart disease tested with 48-hour Holter monitoring]. *Pol Merkuriusz Lek* 2000; 9(50):528–530.

Poldermans D, Fioretti PM, Boersma E, Cornel JH, Borst F, Vermeulen EG et al. Dobutamine-atropine stress echocardiography and clinical data for predicting late cardiac events in patients with suspected coronary artery disease. *Am J Med* 1994; 97(2):119–125.

Scuteri A, Bos AJ, Zonderman AB, Brant LJ, Lakatta EG, Fleg JL. Is the apoE4 allele an independent predictor of coronary events? *Am J Med* 2001; 110(1): 28–32.

Ueda K, Takahashi M, Ozawa K, Kinoshita M. Decreased soluble interleukin-6 receptor in patients with acute myocardial infarction. *Am Heart J* 1999; 138(5 Pt 1):908–915.

Wackers FJ, Brown KA, Heller GV, Kontos MC, Tatum JL, Udelson JE et al. American Society of Nuclear Cardiology position statement on radionuclide imaging in patients with suspected acute ischemic syndromes in the emergency department or chest pain center. *J Nucl Cardiol* 2002; 9(2):246–250.

Index